Weight Training for Women

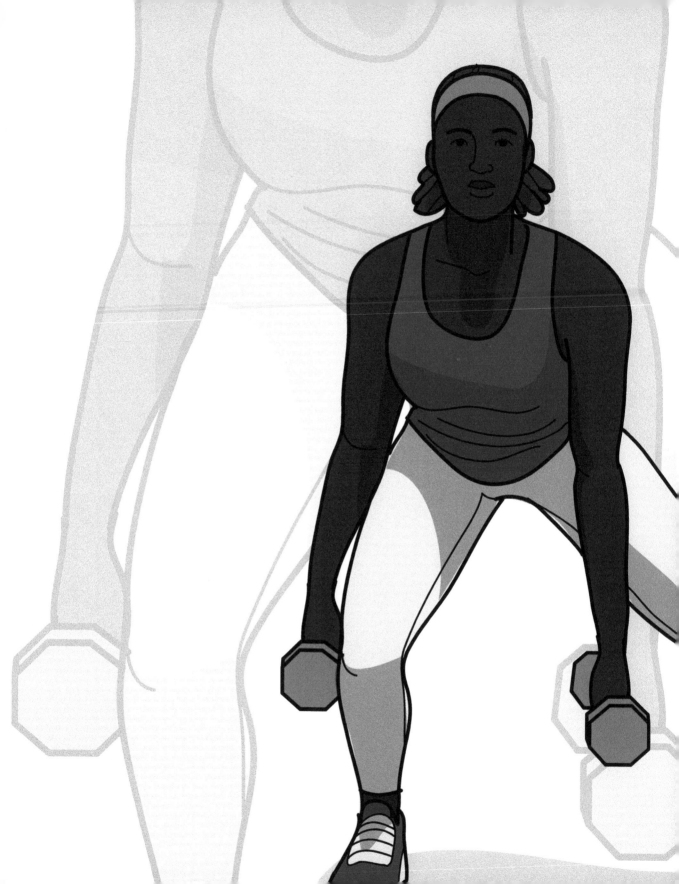

WEIGHT TRAINING
FOR WOMEN

Exercises and Workout Programs
for Building Strength with Free Weights

BRITTANY NOELLE
ILLUSTRATIONS BY CHARLIE LAYTON

ROCKRIDGE
PRESS

To all the followers of @b_noellefitness who have asked for assistance with weightlifting. This is for you!

Interior and Cover Designer: Darren Samuel
Art Producer: Samantha Ulban
Editor: Rachelle Cihonski

Production Editor: Nora Milman
Illustrations by © 2020 Charlie Layton.

ISBN: Print 978-1-64152-738-5 | eBook 978-1-64152-739-2

R0

CONTENTS

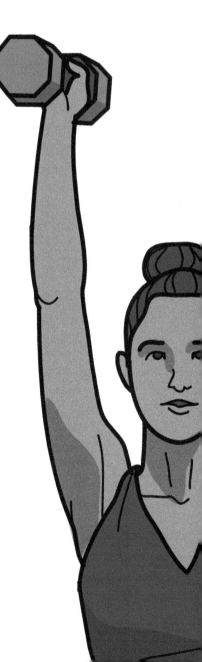

INTRODUCTION

I started running track when I was 7 years old. My first experience with track and field was terrible. I was an awkward, skinny sprinter. Over the years, I became a much better technical sprinter and ended up running in college at UCLA. At the collegiate level, all students were required to go to weightlifting practice, as well as practice on the track. I learned a lot about powerlifting at this time and started to really like lifting weights. Since I was still much skinnier than my teammates, I worked hard to put on extra mass so that I could be more competitive. I also was getting tired of being made fun of by the other students for being too small and "not curvy." I started to see results much faster in the gym than what I was seeing on the track. Getting faster with each workout was very difficult for me, but lifting heavier weight at each practice was fairly easy. This motivated me to keep showing up and adding more weight to the bar with each practice. I knew it would be difficult for me to gain muscle mass; however, I stuck with it and eventually gained the muscle mass I desired over many years of consistent training. It felt amazing to be able to lift a lot of weight for my small size. I wanted to be stronger than the men at my gym who weren't athletes.

Once I graduated with my degree in physiological science, I decided not to go to graduate school for physical therapy, which was my original intention. I still wanted to learn how to fix and prevent injuries, but I decided to get certified as a personal trainer and learn how to help people in a more practical setting. It was the best decision of my life! Not only did I learn a lot about injury prevention, but I also learned a lot more about functional training in general.

Weightlifting has helped me feel strong and powerful, which are two things I think all women should strive for. That is why I wrote this book. I want to use all the knowledge I've gathered over the years to help women begin their weightlifting journey the correct way. I also want to show women that weightlifting is empowering and won't make you any less feminine. In fact, weightlifting helps enhance your body's natural curves!

Weightlifting is important and a great option for all women—no matter your age, background, or body shape. Once you begin your journey, I have no doubt that you'll continue. The power and strength you'll gain will be a life-changing part of your journey and are truly priceless.

How to Use This Book

This book is intended for those new to weightlifting. Therefore, I'll walk you through developing a weightlifting program by teaching you specific warm-ups, exercises, and stretches for each of the body's major muscle groups. At the end of this book, you will also find sample workout programs. Feel free to take pieces of different programs and mix them together once you understand the movements and are comfortable with the concept of programming.

I've also included helpful tips with every exercise in the book, like how to make a movement easier or more difficult. Take special note of any Home Workout Hack tips, as these tips will provide you with alternative movements that you can do if you are at home and are lacking certain equipment. Another thing to pay close attention to are any Lift Safely tips. These will provide you with any additional notes that you'll need in regard to form, range of motion, and properly executing the movements.

While I will go into more detail on this later in the book, it's worth mentioning here that it's critical to warm up properly before working out. A proper warm-up will help you prepare your muscles for the workout as well as prevent injury. It is equally important to stretch after your workout. There will be warm-up movements and stretches provided for each muscle group in this book. In other words, keep reading and you'll have all the tools necessary to learn how to lift weight safely, effectively, and for life!

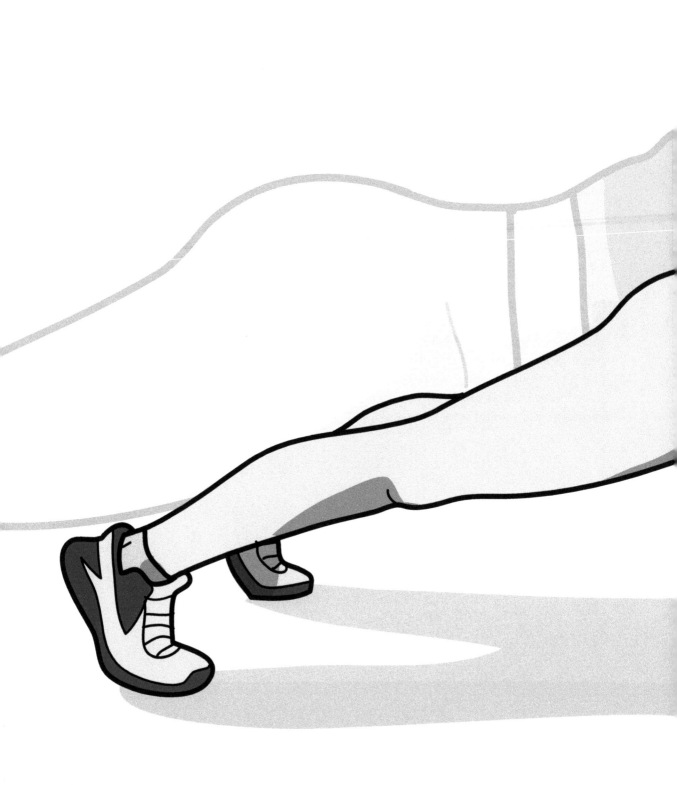

1. PLANNING YOUR PROGRAM

9 Benefits of Weight Training

Why should you begin weightlifting? Appearance aside, there are many physical, mental, and emotional health benefits associated with lifting weights. In addition to improving your strength, an expected benefit most people think of when it comes to weight training, there are numerous other physical benefits, such as increasing bone density, metabolic rate, cognitive ability, coordination and stability, cardiovascular capacity, energy, and cell function, as well as reducing stress. All of these benefits aid in empowering you to feel both physically and mentally strong and help in how you view each day. Below are the details and science supporting each of these impressive benefits.

1. Increased strength. By lifting weights, you will develop the muscle strength necessary for lifting heavier objects inside and outside the gym. Think how much easier tasks like bringing in the groceries and picking up your kids and pets would be with strong muscles! Having stronger muscles will also aid in maintaining an upright posture and supporting your bone structure.

2. Increased bone density. Speaking of bones, many women are at risk of developing osteopenia or osteoporosis—the weakening of your bones with age. Weightlifting can help keep your bones strong as you age by increasing bone density. Working the muscles attached to your bones forces your body to lay down more bone-making materials, which strengthens your bones and increases their density. It's two great benefits in one!

3. Increased metabolic rate. Strength training will also result in you having more overall muscle mass, and the more muscle you have, the more calories you burn at rest. This is because muscle tissue burns more calories. This means you'll burn extra calories even when you're not working out, simply because you have more muscle mass.

4. Increased cognitive ability. Basically, strength training makes you smarter. Your brain has to work differently while strength training. It needs to remember movement patterns, know where your limbs are in relation to your body, and pay attention to the stimuli around you. This is a lot of work for your brain—especially if you are new to weight training. Therefore, it's an excellent way to give your brain a workout. In addition to making you smarter, weightlifting also helps improve your mood and increases your self-esteem, a result of happy hormones (endorphins) being released into your bloodstream.

5. Increased coordination and stability. Lifting weights and coordinating movements help you gain better stability, coordination, and proprioceptive feedback (how your brain recognizes where your body and limbs are when performing movements). This is helpful for preventing you from having clumsy moments or falling.

6. Increased cardiovascular capacity. Weight training may not seem like cardio, but it is when you train at an intensity that raises your heart rate. It's rhythmic in nature, and you repeat the motions of the exercises several times. Also, your heart rate stays increased when you superset exercises—that is, perform movements back-to-back with little to no rest between them. This makes weightlifting a form of cardio (and way less boring than using cardio equipment!).

7. Increased energy. Weightlifting releases hormones in your body that signal your brain to wake up. These happy endorphins give you a natural boost of energy. That's why many people like to weightlift in the morning or during their lunch breaks—to get a little energy boost before starting their day or getting back to work.

8. Better cellular functions. Weightlifting increases the blood lactate concentrations, hemoglobin levels, and capillary-to-fiber ratio in your cells. These increases allow your cells to function more efficiently by causing blood to flow more smoothly throughout the body. With increased blood flow efficiency, oxygen and nutrient delivery to the muscles increases and creates optimal cellular performance.

9. Stress reduction. Weightlifting helps you relieve stress by giving your brain and body a way to externalize any pent-up emotions. The hormones released when you work out help your body counteract the stress-causing hormone cortisol. In addition, with weightlifting, you build confidence and self-esteem, which also reduce stress. So not only do you get to throw some weight around to feel better and relieve tension, but you also get a nice dose of stress-relieving hormones to relax your brain and improve your confidence post-workout.

Identify Your Goals

Now that you know some of the awesome benefits of working out, it's time for you to decide on a goal. Setting a goal drives personal motivation and satisfaction. First and foremost, you need to start by picking a goal that is deeply rooted in your "WHY." Your WHY is something that is very important to you. It isn't something superficial or shallow. Rather, your WHY is something that has a personal emotional trigger associated with it—a deep internal motivation that is unique to you. If your goal doesn't have a WHY attached to it, then you will be less likely to succeed at it. Furthermore, you have to want to achieve that goal for yourself, not because someone else gave you a goal.

The next step is to make sure that your goal is SMART—that means it is Specific, Measurable, Attainable, Realistic, and Time sensitive. For example, a SMART goal could be "I want to lose 10 pounds in 2 months so that I can participate in more activities on our upcoming family vacation. I'm going to achieve this by weightlifting 3 times a week." Losing 10 pounds in 2 months is very specific, measurable, and attainable within the time frame established. It's also realistic that this person can weightlift 3 times a week. Now, to take the SMART goal a step further, the WHY associated with it could be "I want to participate in more activities on vacation because I don't want to be left out of the family photos or miss out on building memories as a family." That WHY has a strong emotion associated with it; therefore, this person is much more likely to lose the 10 pounds, since they decided on this goal for themselves as opposed to someone else deciding on it for them.

When and How Often to Work Out

When and how often to work out really depends on your goals and lifestyle. The important thing is to decide on a routine and stick with it. Check your schedule and realistically determine how many days a week you can commit to working out. Decide if mornings, afternoons, or evenings are best for you based on your schedule and energy levels throughout the day. You may even decide that switching up the time of day works best for you. It will not affect the results of your program, as long as you are consistent about working out for the number of days you commit to. Two days of working out a week is the minimum amount you will need to commit to in order to see changes in your body. At least 3 days is optimal, but some people can handle doing 4 or 5 days depending on their style of working out and goals. You might want to consider starting with fewer days and adding more as you build your workout program. Being aggressive and starting with too many days can lead to unrealistic self-expectations and harm your motivation.

You should plan for your workouts to last anywhere from 30 to 90 minutes, including your warm-up and cooldown. Your goals will determine the length of your weightlifting program. If your goal is to burn fat or lose weight, then you should create circuits of 3 or 4 exercises that you do one after another for one set. This type of workout will include fewer rest breaks and will take less time. If you are trying to put on muscle mass, then your workout will focus on one exercise at a time or supersets with maximum rest and recovery times. This type of workout will take longer and may include more exercises to fatigue a particular muscle group. Another factor that will affect your workout time is the number of days that you commit to working out. If, for example, you're working out 4 or 5 times a week, then 30- to 45-minute intervals would be a good amount of time to help prevent overtraining. (Overtraining happens when you are working out too much and not getting the proper amount of recovery time.) If you are only able to work out 2 or 3 times a week, then 60 to 90 minutes would be ideal to maximize results, since you are committing to fewer days.

WARM-UP BEST PRACTICES

Warming up is an important part of the weightlifting process. You need to make sure that your muscles have proper blood flow and your joints are sufficiently lubricated and mobile before loading them with additional weight. This will make your weightlifting sessions more effective and also prevent injuries from occurring. Here are three best practices for making the most of your warm-up.

- **Warm the muscles you'll be working.** What you include in your warm-up should be based on what you plan to do as a workout that day. For example, if you are working your upper body, then you should include movements that use your arms, such as jumping jacks, bear crawls, or Planks (page 104). If you are working your lower body, then you would include movements like lunges, squats, toe touches, and Butt Kickers (page 48). In the exercise chapters to come, you will see some suggested warm-up movements you can use to prepare those specific muscles to work.
- **Start to elevate your heart rate.** Your warm-up should take anywhere from 5 to 10 minutes. By the end of it, you want to feel like you have a light sweat going. You should also have an elevated heart rate at this point, somewhere around 115 to 125 beats per minute (bpm). Using cardio equipment, such as jogging or walking on an incline on the treadmill, can certainly aid in your warm-up. However, you still want to include a few specific movements to target whatever muscle groups you plan to work that day.
- **Use dynamic movements.** You want your warm-up to be dynamic. This means that you want it to mimic the exercises you plan to do later in your workout—it should serve as movement preparation. For example, standing and reaching toward your toes to stretch your hamstrings is great but not dynamic. A better way to stretch your hamstrings before lifting would be to do walking Straight-Leg Kicks (page 26). The more dynamic a movement is, the more closely it relates to the actions your leg muscles will need to perform to lift effectively.

THE CRITICAL COOLDOWN

Your post-workout cooldown is just as important as your pre-workout warm-up. Just as it is necessary to prepare your muscles and joints for movement, you also need to signal to them that they can relax and move blood to other parts of your body. Pick your cooldown based on what you did for a workout. For example, if you did upper body, then it might be good to passively stretch your back and arms for a few seconds to relieve some of the tension you've built up in them. Passive stretches are great to include in your cooldown. You can hold each stretch for 30 to 45 seconds. You can also use cardio equipment or go for a short walk or very mild jog to cool down.

You do not want to skip your cooldown. Even if you're very tired, it's essential to cool your body down. (Walking to your car or taking a shower does not count.) If you do not, your muscles could experience severe cramping post-workout. Your muscles will also remain in a shortened state, which will negatively impact your joint range of motion and posture.

REST DAYS AND RECOVERY

Rest and recovery are important to take into consideration to maximize your results. If you don't rest and recover, then you'll be at risk of overtraining. The symptoms of overtraining include getting sick, feeling sore, achiness, decreased performance, moodiness, excessive fatigue, insomnia, increased perceived effort during exercise, and injuries.

It is optimal to have at least 2 rest days per week. When you weight train, you break down your muscle tissue. Therefore, your muscles need at least a day to rebuild the muscle fibers stronger than before—this process can sometimes take up to 3 days. You will want to be aware of what muscle groups you are working each day and give each muscle group at least 1 to 2 days to recover. As you progress in your weightlifting journey, you'll become more in tune with your body. When this happens, you'll be able to gauge how much rest and recovery time you need for each muscle group.

Be aware that you will experience some muscle soreness after your first few days of weightlifting. This is called DOMS (delayed-onset muscle soreness). It's the period 24 to 48 hours after weightlifting when your muscles are rebuilding the muscle fibers. The goal is not to be sore after every workout. Eventually, you'll find a balance where you feel worked but not overworked after weightlifting. This also comes with being more in tune with your body as you progress.

6 Tips to Maintain a Life of Lifting

Weightlifting has so many more benefits beyond just aesthetics. While aesthetics may be why you get started or what you hear more about, the other benefits detailed at the start of this chapter can bring so much more to your life. For this reason, you find that you want to make weightlifting a part of your lifestyle. The key to accomplishing this is to find the other motivating factors that keep you connected to a WHY that goes deeper than appearance. Here are a few tips on how to discover those extra motivational factors that will help you maintain a life of lifting.

Tip #1: Don't lift for aesthetics. Looking good is a great way to motivate yourself when you start, but what happens when you get older? As your body starts to change with age, you may not look the same as you did before. If you do, awesome! But it's likely that your ideal aesthetic look won't be manageable long-term. Focus on mastering a particular movement that you couldn't do before or on lifting a specific amount of weight. These types of imperative goals are more motivating to keep you lifting for life than aesthetics alone.

Tip #2: Listen to your body. Weightlifting is great, but it does put a little extra strain on your body, so you want to be smart and listen to your body. Do movements that make your body feel good. Also, rest when your body says that it needs it.

Tip #3: Dedicate time to recovery. As mentioned above, taking care of your body is very important, and there are several things you can do. Spend time stretching and foam rolling every day, or teach yourself other self-myofascial release (SMR) methods. SMR is the process of eliminating knots, or trigger points, in the fascia of your muscles using various massage techniques and tools. Massages are also beneficial to helping your muscles recover, and making sure you get plenty of sleep and water is important.

Tip #4: Get a personal trainer. A personal trainer can help you keep your routine fresh and not boring. They can also program workouts for you to help prevent injury and get the proper rest between workouts. Personal trainers are worth the money. There is no price tag too high on investing in your health.

Tip #5: Switch it up. Mixing up your routine keeps you from getting bored. As you become more confident in weight training, try adding different modalities and equipment, such as kettlebells, TRX (total-body resistance exercise) straps, a ViPR (short for "vitality, performance, and reconditioning"), resistance bands, machines, and cables, into your workout routine. Learning to master movements with new training stimuli will challenge both your brain and body.

Tip #6: Keep it moving. Inspire yourself to do something every day. Make weightlifting a part of your lifestyle, not a chore. A little movement each day helps you maintain what you have—so move it or lose it!

THE FUNDAMENTALS OF LIFTING

There are a handful of basic guidelines for building a solid weightlifting foundation. Keeping these 8 core items in mind whenever you lift weights will help you remain safe and be effective in hitting your goals. Over time, these fundamentals will become second nature to you.

1. **Always engage your core.** No matter what muscle group you're training, your core should be engaged with every movement for stability and safety. To "engage your core" simply means drawing your belly button into the spine. It should be a similar feeling to what you would do if you were planning to blow up a balloon or preparing for someone to poke you in the stomach. As you become a more experienced weightlifter, engaging your core will happen automatically, and you won't need to think about it as often. That said, in each of the exercise chapters, I have included a reminder to engage your core while performing every movement. These reminders are important as you build your program because engaging your core is key to building stability and strength, moving safely, and developing an effective workout.

2. **Never skip warm-up and cooldown.** Always warm up properly before you lift and leave time to cool down when you finish. Warming up is important because it prepares the body for activity. When you warm up, your temperature rises, which results in loosening your joints and increasing blood flow. With loosened joints and increased blood flow, you will create less stress on your joints, which will create more ease in performing exercises. Cooling down is equally important because it reduces heart and breathing rates, which lowers your body temperature. In addition, your muscles return to their resting lengths and your body is then ready for normal activity. When you skip warming up or cooling down, you risk injury or other issues. For example, if you abruptly stop exercising, your heart rate may drop too quickly, which could result in fainting.

3. **Be safe when you are lifting.** Make sure the space around you is open and safe, and there are no free weights lying around or any equipment that you can trip over. Additionally, make sure you have someone around to spot you if you plan on lifting heavier weights than you are used to.

4. **Do not drop your weights.** There's a chance they can rebound and hit you or someone else. Try to control the return of your weights or ask your spotter to assist you if you run out of strength.

5. **Keep recovery in mind.** You don't want to work the same muscle groups two days in a row. If you are planning to do full-body workouts each day, then switch up the plane of movement or modality. For example, if you did Forward Lunges yesterday, then do Lateral Lunges today.

6. **Work in different planes of motion.** This will help keep the muscle groups of your body balanced. It will also ensure that your body is prepared for daily functional movements. The three planes of motion are sagittal, frontal, and transverse. The sagittal plane divides the body into left and right halves. Activities such as walking and running are done in the sagittal plane—in fact, most of us tend to stick to sagittal plane movements. However, it is key to mix up your training to include movements in all three planes in order to keep the body balanced and to avoid injury. The frontal plane divides the body into front and back halves. Movements in the frontal plane include jumping jacks and Lateral Lunges. The transverse plane divides the body into top and bottom halves. The transverse plane includes movements such as twisting (wood chops), swinging (think golfing), and push-ups.

7. **Track your progress.** You can't tell where you're going if you don't know where you came from. Write down your exercises, weight, sets, reps, and rest time for each workout. This will help you keep track of your progress and determine your next set of goals.

8. **Stay hydrated.** Make sure you're properly hydrated before a workout. Also, have water or another proper hydration beverage with you while working out to prevent cramping and feeling light-headed, and to rehydrate post-workout.

The Role of Cardio

Cardio is important to add into your routine if you are looking to lose weight or body fat. There are two main types of cardio: steady state and HIIT (high-intensity interval training). Steady-state cardio is when you maintain a steady and continuous effort in your workout. The recommended time for steady-state cardio is 1 hour for maximum results where you maintain a heart rate of 45 to 50 percent of your maximum heart rate. This could be walking on the treadmill at an incline, using the elliptical or StairMaster, rowing, swimming laps, or going for a hike outside. Wearing a heart rate monitor is really helpful because keeping your heart rate within a certain "fat burning" range is important. The fat-burning range is the heart rate range that is optimal for burning fat, rather than carbohydrates, for fuel.

HIIT is when you do a mix of high-intensity and low-intensity cardio intervals. You can choose various lengths of time for your intervals. For example, intervals can be up to 1 minute each, during which your heart rate will increase to a high "anaerobic" rate, followed by a rest period of 1 minute if you're looking to have a 1:1 work-to-rest ratio for your interval. Another example would be to sprint for 30 seconds and then walk for 1 minute. The sprint is the high-intensity portion, and the walk is the low-intensity portion. You can vary the work-to-rest ratios depending on your goals. Again, having a heart rate monitor can be very helpful for determining these times.

Cardio can still be done if you're working on increasing your muscle mass. However, you want to focus on high-intensity cardio—things like sprinting, sled pushes, or biking with high resistance. These types of explosive movements will help you gain strength and power. When performing these exercises, you need to do 2 to 8 sets of maximum-effort intervals to build strength and power without burning muscle.

A Note on Diet

Let's start by reframing the word "diet" to mean nutrition and eating habits. Nutrition is an important element of achieving your goals. You want to eat foods that promote high energy levels and that have beneficial nutritional value. These foods are going to be fresh and nonprocessed items—typically, what you would find in the outer aisles of the grocery store (think produce and meat) as opposed to the frozen premade food and center aisles. Your goals will determine how much food you should consume. If you want to gain muscle mass, then you'll need to eat more calories than what you burn on a daily basis. If you are trying to lose weight, then you'll need to eat fewer calories than what you burn on a daily basis.

Instead of approaching food with a mind-set of restriction, think of foods as what you want to eat more of, eat some of, or eat less of.

- **Eat MORE** of foods like eggs, fish, chicken, turkey, duck breasts, lean beef, bison, lamb, plain Greek yogurt, tempeh, lentils, beans, whole grains, quinoa, plain kefir, fruits and vegetables, potatoes, olive oil, avocado, olives, nuts, and almond and cashew butters.
- **Eat SOME** of foods like tofu, medium lean meats, edamame, Canadian bacon, meat jerky, poultry sausage, protein powder, white rice, milk, vegetable juice, flavored yogurt, pancakes/waffles, whole-grain crackers, oat-based granola bars, canned/dried fruit, virgin and light olive oil, sesame oil, flaxseed oil, coconut milk, peanut butter, dark chocolate, cream, and flavored nut butters.
- **Eat LESS** of foods like fried foods, high-fat ground meat, processed meat or deli meat, protein bars, high-mercury fish, fruit juices, cereal and cereal bars, sugar, flavored milk, soda, honey, syrups, jellies, pretzels, crackers, chips, pastries, butter, processed cheeses, marinades and dressings containing saturated fats, trans fats, and hydrogenated oils.

PRE-WORKOUT NUTRITION

It is important to be properly fueled before starting your workout. You need enough energy to make it through your workout so that you don't become light-headed or dizzy as a result of low glucose levels from a lack of food. A good rule of thumb is to eat about 2 hours before your workout—that way your body has enough time to digest everything. Your meal should consist of protein, vegetables and fruits (considered fibrous carbohydrates), good fat (like olive oil or avocado), and some complex carbs (such as quinoa or rice). Complex carbs help keep your blood glucose levels stable while you work out. If you don't have time for a full pre-workout meal, opt for a small snack at least 30 minutes prior to training. This snack should ideally combine a carb and protein for optimal energy, like an apple and nut butter or chicken breast, rice, and sweet potato. Additionally, you want to make sure you are well hydrated before your workout. Drink about 16 to 32 ounces of water within that 2-hour window before your workout.

POST-WORKOUT NUTRITION

It is important to fuel your body properly after a workout to maximize muscle repair. Though nutrition is unique to each individual, generally speaking it is best to consume about 25 grams of protein and 25 grams of carbs within 30 to 60 minutes post-workout for optimal results. This is because of the excess post-exercise oxygen consumption state that your body will be in post-workout, due to the number of calories you burned as a result of weightlifting. Consuming this amount of protein can be done by having a protein shake; however, it's best to consume whole foods if you can. A good carb source like vegetables or fruits would suffice, as you do not need as hearty of a carb as you did pre-workout. Although it is optimal to eat within 30 to 60 minutes post-workout, don't stress if you need to eat a little later due to not being hungry or not having the time. New research shows that your body is breaking down muscle and rebuilding it all day after weightlifting. Therefore, as long as you consume the necessary amount of protein and carbs for recovery, the time doesn't matter for most people. Remember that your pre- and post-workout nutrition is going to vary slightly with your goals. Consult a dietitian if you are in need of a specific nutrition plan.

Tracking Your Progress

As mentioned earlier, tracking your progress is important for making sure that you are on target to achieving your goals. You should track both your food and your workouts to make sure that you are making progress. A few good ways to track these are by writing them down in a workout journal, creating a spreadsheet on your computer, taking notes on your phone, or using a fitness app. A nutrition app like MyFitnessPal is prepopulated with popular food and restaurants, so you can see how many calories you've consumed throughout the day. Most fitness trackers, such as Fitbit, Garmin, and Apple Watch, have workout tracking capabilities, providing additional motivation to hit your goals. They are great for monitoring your vitals and also for sharing your progress with friends and family for some group support. The more ways you have of holding yourself accountable, the more successful you'll be at reaching your goals and seeing results.

Speaking of accountability, you can also have an online personal trainer send you workouts digitally via apps like Trainerize. This is great for having a weekly custom program sent to you and for tracking your progress. There are many top-notch trainers to choose from, and the app is easily accessed from your phone, tablet, or computer.

If you would prefer to write down your workouts as opposed to using an app, make sure you include the number of reps, sets, time rested, tempo, and weight used. If you are tracking your food manually, then simply write down what you eat and the portion size throughout the day. Taking photos of your food is another great way to manage what you eat. It's also great data to share with your dietitian or trainer when they ask for your food log.

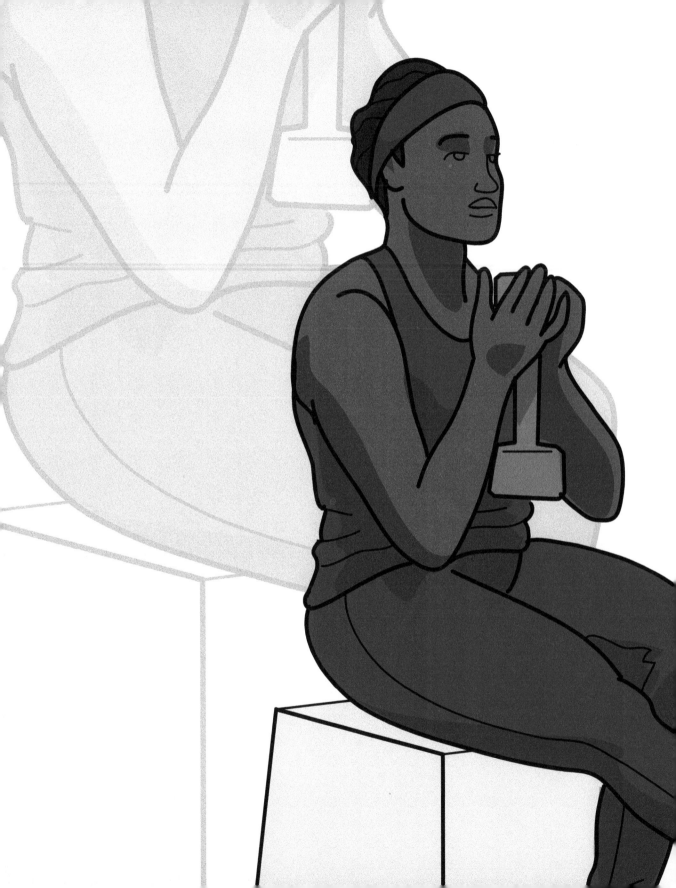

2. EQUIPMENT AND ENVIRONMENT

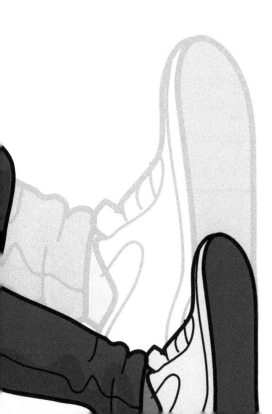

This chapter will focus on the things to consider when evaluating your workout environment and equipment options. Depending on your goals and schedule, you may opt for home workouts and need information on what you'll need at home to create your personal gym. If you feel a trainer and/or a dedicated fitness space may help you stay motivated, you might choose to work out in a gym, where a trainer can meet you at regularly scheduled times. To help you feel prepared and confident for a gym experience, we will review what to expect, proper protocol, and clothing options. Do you know the differences between free weights and machines? We will look at which equipment is best for helping you with your program and why. Overall, we'll explore the things you'll want to consider in making these decisions so that you can be safe and have an effective weightlifting program.

Gym vs. Home Workouts

Feel intimidated weightlifting in a gym? No worries, that's a normal feeling to have. This book will teach you everything you need to know so that you can walk over to the weight rack with confidence and a workout plan in hand.

There are a few key differences between working out at a gym versus at home. The first is the selection of equipment. The gym offers a large variety of weightlifting and cardio equipment, which is important as you progress through your program and need heavier weights. You will have multiple sets of dumbbells, kettlebells, barbells, resistance bands, cables, and machines at your disposal. You will also have access to heavier weights with safety mechanisms, such as a leg press machine, and a weightlifting rack where you can complete powerlifting movements. This type of equipment allows you to lift much heavier weights than you can at home because of the safety of the rack. It may sound like too much to consider and makes this all feel intimidating, but all these options are valuable because they give you more freedom to select what works best for you and your body. Something else to consider about the gym is that there are trainers who can demonstrate proper usage of the equipment as well as watch you to make sure you're using the equipment correctly.

The gym is also a great motivator because you have to make an effort and physically go there as opposed to staying in your home. Some people find that if they schedule gym time like they do other activities, and they're not home being distracted, they are more apt to be consistent with their workouts. In addition, when you're at the gym, you are around other people and more likely to push yourself.

If after reading this book you are still feeling a little hesitant about lifting weights at the gym, take baby steps. Start by grabbing a few weights and find a corner in the gym to do your workout. If your gym has a studio for classes, the studio is a more private place to work out when there isn't a class in session. If you're still not able to go to the gym, this book includes plenty of Home Workout Hack tips that will aid you in getting the most out of your program while at home.

There are downsides to using a gym. At times, there are lines to use the equipment and you may need to wait for someone else to finish using a piece of equipment that you want to use. In addition, while most gyms are fairly clean, you may find that with continual, nonstop use, some of the equipment handles and seats need to be wiped down between uses. At home, there is never a line for equipment, and everything is always clean and ready for your use. But while a home gym may sound ideal, keep in mind that you will likely have less variety of equipment available to you and you'll need to continue to purchase heavier weights as you progress in your weightlifting program.

Whichever you choose, you need to find the best way to maximize your program. The most important thing is that you commit to yourself and stick with it no matter where you are.

The Weights

There are basically two types of weights to consider: free weights and machines. Free weights are any type of weight that you can use freely in all planes of motion. Simply put, they aren't attached to anything, so you have full control over them. The advantage to using free weights is that they are the most functional pieces of equipment, meaning they allow you to move in the same ways that you do in real life when you are going about your daily activities. Free weights help your muscles develop under different lines of stress, which is essential for injury prevention and better overall movement. You also need to be more careful with free weights *because* you have complete control over them. Therefore, there is nothing to protect you if you use the weights with incorrect form. Machines are in fixed positions. You can only push or pull the weight in a particular line of stress and in a particular motion. This is safer but not functional. You rarely do anything in real life that allows your body to move in a straight line along a single plane. This means that you could put yourself at risk for injury even when using a machine, because your anatomical structure and natural way of moving may not align with the machines.

All of the exercises listed in the book will use free weights so that the exercises can easily be done at the gym or in a home gym setting. In addition, free weights allow the exercise measurements to remain constant, which is important for tracking your progress. You need to know how much weight you are lifting at all times so that you can accurately record your progress. We will discuss the types of free weights used in this book in the following sections. Keep in mind that most of the exercises in this book can be done utilizing either type of free weight.

DUMBBELLS

Dumbbells are short bars with weights at each end. Dumbbells can be used individually or as pairs. This will allow you to work each arm independently of the other (or unilateral training). This is great for making sure that one arm isn't overcompensating for the other and that your muscles are well balanced. Another benefit of using dumbbells is that you can position them in a way that best suits your joints, like holding them closer or farther away from your body based on what's comfortable to you. You can also rotate the dumbbells internally and externally to adjust for comfort. Additionally, dumbbells are easier to drop if you absolutely must while performing an exercise. You should never drop your weights, especially as you're shifting between exercises. However, if you don't have a spotter and you've fatigued your muscles to failure, it's safer to drop the weights than to risk injury by holding on to the dumbbells. If you must drop the weights, always be sure you are in an open space and that you won't hurt anyone else.

BARBELLS

Barbells, on the other hand, have a longer metal bar with weight disks on each end. Some barbells allow you to adjust the amount of weight on each end. Other barbells are a fixed weight, like with dumbbells. Barbells are great for loading when doing leg exercises. ("Loading" is a common term for adding more weight to a movement.) Since women tend to have more strength in their lower bodies as opposed to their upper bodies, it's easier to use heavier weights with barbells because the weight is being supported with your shoulders and upper back instead of just with your arms. Also, barbells sometimes feel easier to use because you grip with both hands; therefore, you are able to better stabilize yourself when performing pushing and pulling movements. On the negative side, barbells can allow you to compensate by pushing more with one side than the other, so be aware of that. Additionally, barbells are a little more cumbersome to have around the house and a little awkward to maneuver. Once you get the hang of barbells, however, they're a great resource, especially for exercises where you want to use heavier weight. You can use dumbbells instead of barbells for exercises, but then you run the risk of losing your grip before completing your set. When this happens, you will likely need to place your dumbbells down before continuing on with the movement, which is not ideal.

GYM ETIQUETTE

Gym etiquette is very important if you want to maintain a positive gym environment. No one wants to lift with the woman who doesn't follow the rules. Don't be *that* woman! Here are a few things to keep in mind.

Don't hog equipment. Everyone is trying to get their workouts in with limited equipment and time. Complete your set and then allow someone else to work with the equipment during your rest period. Sharing is caring!

Clean up after yourself. Just like sharing, other common kindergarten rules apply at the gym, including returning equipment to its original spot. Rerack your weights and wipe everything down, including anything that may have made contact with your sweat, like benches, chairs, balls, handles, and cardio equipment.

Don't talk on your phone. No one wants to hear your latest gossip while they're trying to focus on their workout. Take your conversation out to the lobby. Texting is appropriate, but be mindful of how long you're sitting on equipment while doing it. Two minutes is enough time to rest. Anything longer and you should vacate the machine or bench and let someone else use it.

Ask to work in with someone. Don't just commandeer someone's weights or machine without asking them. If you'd like to use a piece of equipment that someone else is using, politely ask how many sets they have left. Then either wait for them to finish or ask to work in (use the weight or equipment while they rest) with them.

Practice good hygiene. Make sure to wear fresh gym clothes and take the proper measures to prevent odor once you start sweating by refreshing your deodorant or antiperspirant before your workout. A good rule of thumb is that if you can smell yourself, then others can probably smell you, too. Also, have a towel with you to wipe off excess sweat from yourself or equipment that you come into contact with. The gym is a much nicer place when everyone practices good hygiene.

CONTINUED ▶

▶ CONTINUED

Don't make it awkward for others. The gym is oftentimes filled with good-looking people with great bodies. However, they are there to work out just like you are. Be friendly, but remember to treat the gym more or less like a place of work, not a club.

Respect other people's workouts. It's perfectly fine to gain inspiration from another member's or a trainer's workout. However, don't copy everything that someone else is doing in a workout. You don't know their goals, and if they're a professional, then you're stealing their workout. It's much nicer to go up to the person when they're free and ask if they would mind assisting you in creating some of your own workouts. You can also ask them to explain the benefits of the exercise you were thinking of copying.

Clothing and Other Gear

Typically, women wear leggings or shorts to the gym to allow for dynamic movements. Sweatpants are perfectly fine, too, though you may find yourself uncomfortably hot. Choose bottoms designed for working out so that they are moisture wicking and breathable to prevent discomfort or, worse, an infection. (Cotton underwear is also suggested for that reason.) Wear a supportive sports bra and a moisture-wicking top as well. You can choose a tank top or a short-sleeve or long-sleeve shirt, depending on your comfort level. Recommended fabrics for tops and bottoms include polyester, nylon, spandex, and cotton.

It is also recommended that you wear athletic sneakers. A sneaker designed for cross-training would be best, as opposed to a running shoe or a casual sneaker. You want the shoe to be supportive and relatively flat to allow for stability and dynamic movement while weightlifting. It's best to go to an athletic store and try on a few different brands to find out what's best for you. Everyone's feet are different, so try on your first pair of sneakers and do a few dynamic movements such as walking, jumping, and squatting. You may also need insoles to correct any imbalances in your feet.

In terms of additional items, there are a few things you should consider. Weight gloves are useful for keeping your hands from developing calluses and for improving grip strength. It is also a good idea to have a water bottle with you to stay hydrated during your workout, as well as a towel or two to wipe off sweat and to lay on communal equipment. It is also useful to bring a small drawstring bag with you to the gym to place all these items in to avoid cluttering up the gym floor.

Setting Up a Home Gym

If you prefer to train at home rather than in a gym, I recommend acquiring a set of dumbbells and a barbell in order to do the workout movements in this book. Look for a dumbbell set that allows you to change the weight rather than a set with a fixed weight, so that way you only need one set instead of multiples. The same rule applies to purchasing a barbell—try to find one that allows you to add and remove weight plates so that you can better maximize your space. It is a good idea to purchase iron dumbbells and barbells if you plan to keep your weights outside, because they hold up better in harsh weather. You can get the colorful neoprene weights for indoor use.

If you have the space, it would also be helpful for you to have a weight bench. Other pieces of equipment to consider purchasing are a foam roller, a stability ball, resistance bands, a medicine ball, ankle weights, booty bands, a yoga mat, and a step. (You can purchase a kit of resistance bands that allow you to change out the handles, creating multiple resistance options. This is useful for conserving space, similar to the suggestion above for dumbbells and barbells.) Decide what to purchase based on what you feel is appropriate for your fitness level. All of the equipment is very useful and will maximize your home weightlifting experience. You can purchase any of this equipment online, which is great because then it's delivered straight to your front door. While online, you may want to look for gym storage ideas to help keep your equipment organized and out of your way.

When setting up your workout space, choose a place with good lighting and a mirror, if possible, so that you can check your form as you move. You want to have plenty of open space for dynamic movements, as you don't want to accidentally step on anything or knock something over. Carpet is nice so that you have extra padding for floor exercises; it's also a good way to deaden the noise when putting the weights down. However, keep in mind that carpet will be more unstable (which will make movements more challenging), and it's harder to clean sweat off a carpet. I would recommend an easy-to-clean rubber floor installed specifically for your home gym. This type of floor is stable, has some give to it to help absorb the impact of more explosive movements, and it's easy to clean. Wooden floors are adequate, but it is recommended that you put something between the floor and the weights to avoid scratches.

Some people enjoy listening to music while they work out, so consider putting a stereo system in your home gym. It may also be good to have a water source to refill your water bottle during your workouts. A fan or portable heater may also be necessary for keeping the gym at an ideal temperature while working out.

All things considered, the cost of a home gym depends on how much equipment you want and how much functional space you'd like to have. You may start with a simple investment of $50 for a few weights to get started. Investing in a full set of free weights could cost as much as $500. As you progress, you may want to invest in some cardio equipment for your home gym as well. This could bring your cost closer to $2,000 in total. Start small with an initial investment and then add more equipment as your passion for weightlifting grows.

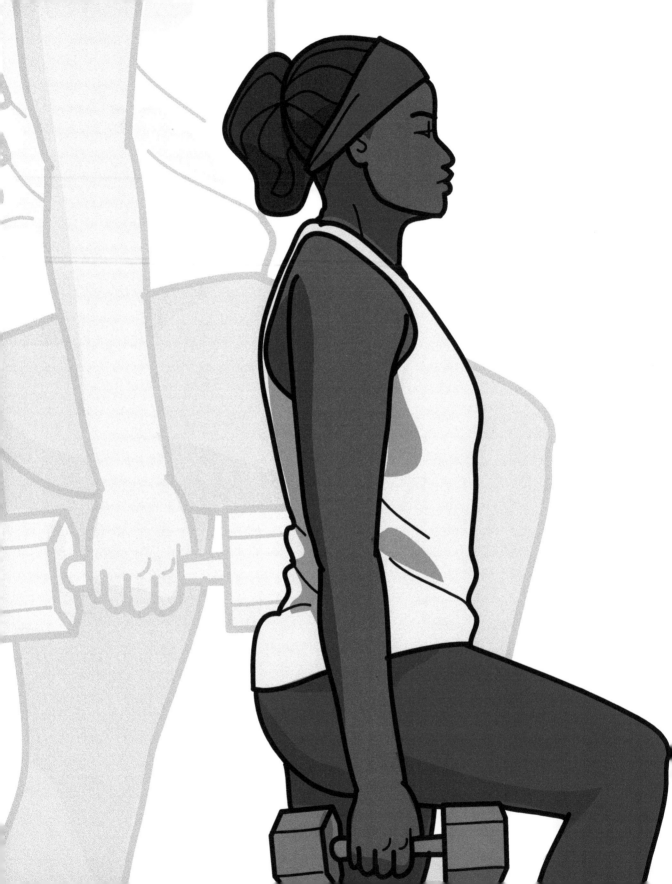

3. GLUTES AND HAMSTRINGS

The glutes are the muscles that make up your buttocks and work as stabilizers for your pelvis while performing movements such as walking and standing. They also help with movements like outwardly rotating the thigh. The muscles that make up this group include the gluteus maximus, gluteus medius, and gluteus minimus.

The hamstrings are the muscles that run along the backs of your thighs. The muscles that make up this group are the semimembranosus, semitendinosus, and biceps femoris. This muscle group is responsible for hip extension and knee flexion (bending your knee). You use your hamstrings for movements like stepping up and running.

It's important to note that the glutes and hamstrings are also two of the muscle groups that make up your core. (Your core is not just comprised of your abdominals, as is commonly believed. The core includes any muscle that helps sync actions between your upper and lower halves.) Because you use these muscles for daily activities, it's important to prepare them adequately in order to avoid injury or strain. You need to spend extra time warming them up pre-workout and stretching them post-workout.

People often think that they have "tight" hamstrings and that they need to stretch them more, but actually, this is not the case for most people. People who sit for long periods of time experience shortness in the muscles of the hips, lower back, and glutes. Shortness means that the muscle fibers remain in a shortened or contracted state after prolonged sitting. As a result, the pelvis becomes rotated in a way that causes the hamstrings to be lengthened. Therefore, the feeling that most people associate with tightness is actually the feeling of being taut—the muscle has lengthened to its full capacity and has no more room for movement. To prevent this, consider doing movements that will stretch the hips and engage the glutes as opposed to overstretching the hamstrings, such as the Pretzel Stretch in this chapter (page 42).

Before You Lift:

Remember to keep your core engaged while executing the movements in this chapter. You can also perform each of these movements in front of a mirror, or record yourself, to double-check your form.

STRAIGHT-LEG KICK

Straight-Leg Kicks are often referred to as Frankenstein or monster kicks because of the resemblance to the fictional character when performing this movement. It's a great movement for actively stretching the hamstrings and warming up the core.

1. Stand with your feet hip-width apart.

2. Take a step forward with your left leg as you kick your right leg into the air and attempt to touch your toes with your left hand.

3. Return to the starting position and then step forward with your right leg, kicking your left leg into the air and reaching for your toes with your right hand.

4. Repeat this movement until you feel warmed up, moving forward as you alternate kicking your legs in front of you. You should feel and look like Frankenstein's monster when performing this movement.

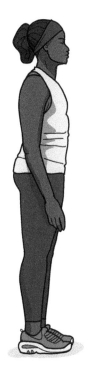

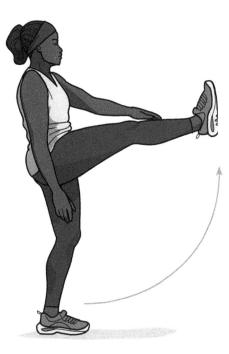

WORLD'S GREATEST STRETCH

This stretch is ideal for increasing range of motion in the hip joint, increasing mobility, and providing a dynamic stretch for the hamstrings. In addition, it warms up your upper body and core. This is why it's called the World's Greatest Stretch—it stretches so many muscle groups at one time.

1. Stand with your feet hip-width apart. Hinge from your hips and reach your hands down to the ground. Try to touch the ground without bending your knees so that you feel a nice stretch in your hamstrings.

2. Once the palms of your hands are on the ground, walk them forward until you are in a push-up position. If you're not able to place your palms on the ground, bend your knees slightly to help you reach. Your hips and shoulders should be aligned.

3. Take your left foot forward and place it on the ground on the outside of your left hand. Press your right hand into the floor as you lift your left hand into the air, rotating through your thoracic spine to open your chest toward your left side. Follow your hand with your eyes.

4. Return your hand to the floor, then return your foot to the starting push-up position.

5. Take your right foot forward and place it on the ground on the outside of your right hand, and repeat the twist on the opposite side.

6. Return to the push-up position. Walk your hands back toward your feet as you raise your hips and attempt to keep your legs straight and heels down, making your way back up to a standing position.

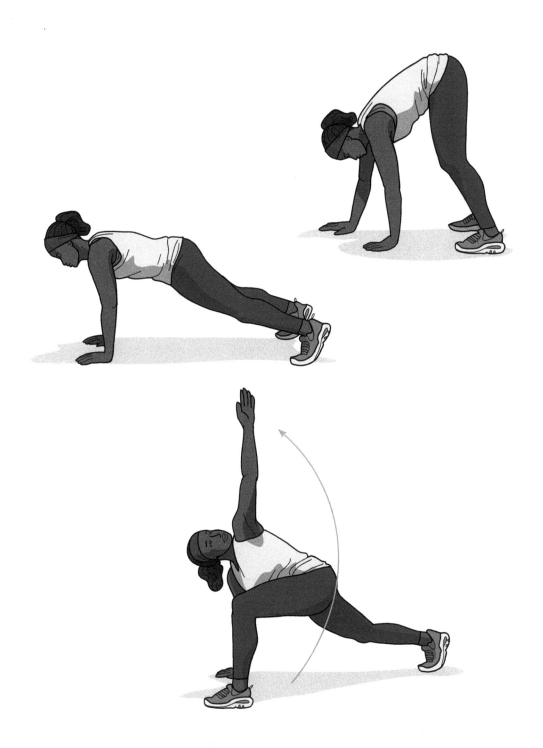

DEADLIFT

ADDITIONAL MUSCLES WORKED: *Back, Core*

This complex movement engages muscle groups in the upper and lower parts of the body. It's also great for core development and neurological coordination.

1. Stand with your feet hip-width apart and toes facing forward, holding dumbbells or a barbell in your hands.

2. Hinge from your hips and push your butt back like you're trying to get it to touch an imaginary wall behind you. Keep your knees soft, but do not bend them, to engage the hamstrings. Keep your back flat and shoulder blades squeezed together to engage your upper back muscles as you reach and move the weights toward your shins. Do not round or hyperextend your back.

3. Once you hit your end range of motion (as low as you can get without rounding your back), squeeze your glutes to drive your hips forward and return to the upright standing position.

Lift Safely: This exercise should only be felt in your hamstrings and glutes. Should you experience any lower back pain, abandon the weights and work only on the hip-hinging pattern.

Make It Easier: Feel free to play around with the position of your feet. You may need a wider (or narrower) stance to keep your spine from rounding at the end position of the Deadlift. You may also need to turn your feet out slightly (so your toes point out) to achieve the ideal position for your body.

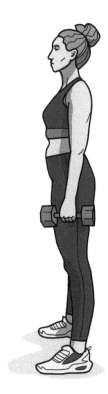

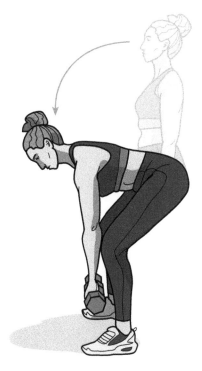

SINGLE-LEG ROMANIAN DEADLIFT

ADDITIONAL MUSCLES WORKED: *Back, Core*

This movement works the same group of muscles as the Deadlift but adds a layer of complexity by challenging your balance. It also helps fix any imbalances between your left and right halves.

1. Stand with your feet hip-width apart and hold a dumbbell or barbell in front of you with both hands, elbows straight, and the weight close to your body. (Almost as if you plan to scrape your shins with the weight on the way down.)

2. Hinge from your hips, keeping your elbows straight, and lift one foot off the ground as you lower your chest and the weight down toward your shins, allowing your leg to come up behind you. Think about kicking your heel to the sky and flex your toes toward your shin as you kick your leg back. (You want your shoulders and foot to move at the same time, like a pendulum.) Do not attempt to bring the weight to the floor. Stop once you feel your spine start to round.

3. Return to the upright starting position. You may place your foot down between reps to regain your balance if you need to.

4. Repeat on the opposite leg.

Lift Safely: Keep your back flat and your hips square to the ground; avoid opening up at the hip. You want to really feel your glutes and hamstrings working during this exercise. If any discomfort is felt in your back, abandon the weights, and make adjustments to your form.

Make It Easier: Tap your foot on the ground in between reps.

Home Workout Hack: Place a broomstick on your back and try to maintain contact between the broom and your neck, mid back, and butt as you perform the movement with no weight. This will help you learn the proper spinal alignment for this movement.

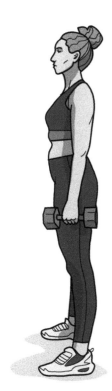

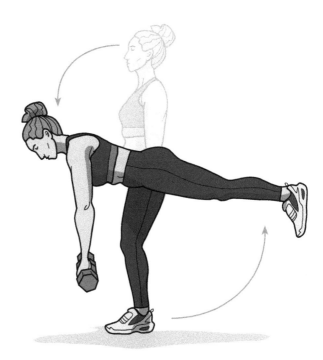

GLUTE BRIDGE

ADDITIONAL MUSCLES WORKED: *Core*

This exercise is very effective in building and toning your glutes and hamstrings. It is also an easier movement to master than Deadlifts.

1. Lie on your back with the bottom of your feet on the floor, hip-width apart, and your toes facing forward.

2. Place a dumbbell or barbell on your hips just below your hip bones and hold it there.

3. Drive out of your heels and squeeze your glutes to lift your hips off the ground while keeping your head and shoulders down and relaxed. Hold at the top of the bridge for 2 seconds.

4. Return your hips to the ground.

Lift Safely: Use your glutes to initiate this movement and not your lower back. Make sure that as you perform this exercise, your knees track over your ankles. Do not let them cave inward or fall outward.

Make It Harder: Use a weight bench or a plyo box to perform barbell hip thrusters. Sit with your shoulder blades in contact with the bench and your feet hip-width apart, toes facing forward. Place the bar across your hips with a pad. Lift your hips off the ground and squeeze your glutes at the top. Keep your shoulders in contact with the bench throughout the movement and your head up with neck relaxed. Lower your hips back down and follow the movement with your shoulders so that you move as one unit.

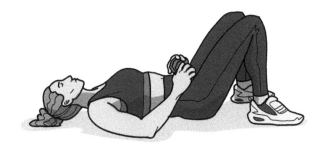

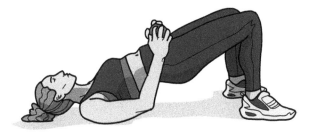

SINGLE-LEG GLUTE BRIDGE

ADDITIONAL MUSCLES WORKED: *Core, Hip Flexors*

This is a more difficult progression from a standard Glute Bridge. The single-leg nature of this movement makes you engage your core and glutes more, compared to performing the movement with both legs.

1. Lie on your back with the bottom of your feet on the floor, hip-width apart, and your toes facing forward.

2. Place a dumbbell or barbell on your hips just below your hip bones and hold it there.

3. Lift one foot off the ground and up to the sky. Squeeze the glutes of the leg on the floor and push with the grounded heel to bring your hips up into a bridge. Hold for about 2 seconds before lowering your hips back down to the ground.

4. You can do all the repetitions on one leg or alternate legs.

Lift Safely: Make sure your knee tracks over your ankle throughout the movement. Don't hyperextend your back at the top of the bridge. Use only your glutes to propel the movement, not your lower back.

Make It Easier: Reduce the range of motion of the exercise by not driving your hips as high. If needed, abandon the weights and perform this movement with body weight.

Make It Harder: Use a heavier weight. You can also drop the elevated leg to the side a few inches and then return it to the center for each repetition. This will challenge your core stability even more.

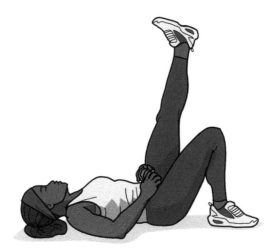

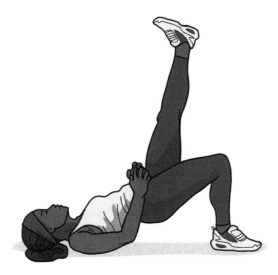

STEP-UP

ADDITIONAL MUSCLES WORKED: *Core, Hip Flexors, Quads*

This movement is great for strengthening the glutes and hamstrings while also improving your balance and stability. Additionally, it will improve your ability to walk up and down stairs.

1. Find a stable chair, bench, step, or box to step on. The surface should be 6 to 18 inches off the floor, depending on your height and skill level.

2. If you have dumbbells, hold those at your sides or hold one at your chest with both hands. If you have a barbell, then place it behind your neck, resting on your shoulders.

3. Stand in front of the chair or box and place your right foot on it.

4. Drive up through your right leg to stand as you bring your left leg up so that your left knee forms a 90-degree angle in front of you at hip height. Squeeze your right glute at the end range of the movement.

5. Reverse the movement and step back onto the floor with both feet.

6. You can repeat this motion on the right leg and then switch to the left, or alternate between legs for each repetition.

Lift Safely: Keep an eye on your knee as you perform your Step-Ups. Your knee should track above your ankle throughout the movement (meaning it doesn't cave in or out). Also, keep your knee behind your toes as you step up, and try your best to not allow your knee to move too far past your toes on the way down. Land softly and double-check that there is nothing in your path to step on as you come down.

Make It Harder: Each Step-Up should be one fluid motion, without pausing in the middle. This will test your balance.

Home Workout Hack: If you are having trouble finding a stable chair for your Step-Ups, try looking around your home for other stable surfaces, like stairs in the house, your outdoor patio, or even a stable step stool.

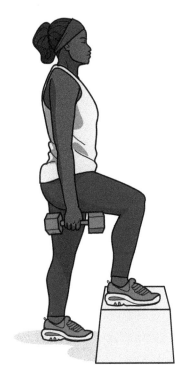

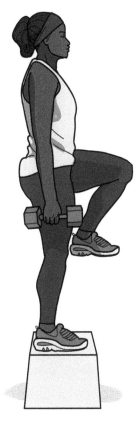

LATERAL STEP-UP

ADDITIONAL MUSCLES WORKED: *Core, Hip Flexors, Quads*

This movement will challenge your inner and outer thigh muscles more than the previous Step-Ups, while also promoting great glute activation.

1. Find a stable chair, bench, step, or box to step on. The surface should be 6 to 18 inches off the floor, depending on your height and skill level.

2. If you have dumbbells, hold those at your sides or hold one at your chest with both hands. If you have a barbell, then place it behind your neck, resting on your shoulders.

3. Stand next to the box, chair, or step so it is on your left side.

4. Keeping the box or step on your left side, step laterally onto the box with your left foot as you bring your right leg up and drive your knee to hip height, knee bent to a 90-degree angle. Squeeze your glutes at the top.

5. Step down and take your foot completely off the box or step before repeating the movement. Perform all the reps on this side before repeating on the opposite side.

Lift Safely: Keep an eye on your knee as you perform your Step-Ups. Your knee should track above your ankle throughout the movement (meaning it doesn't cave in or out). Also, keep your knee behind your toes as you step up, and try your best to not allow your knee to move too far past your toes on the way down. Land softly and double-check that there is nothing in your path to step on as you come down.

Make It Harder: Each Step-Up should be one fluid motion, without pausing in the middle. This will test your balance.

Home Workout Hack: If you are having trouble finding a stable chair for your step-ups, try looking around your home for other stable surfaces, like stairs in the house, your outdoor patio, or even a stable step stool.

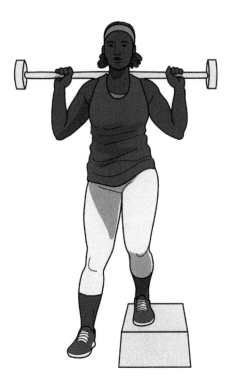

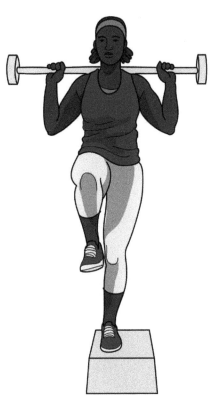

PRETZEL STRETCH

This stretch is perfect for stretching the glute muscles without overstretching the hamstrings.

1. Sit on the ground in a cross-legged position.

2. Place your left foot on the outside of your right knee.

3. Take your right arm and place your left knee in the crease of your right elbow. Sit up as tall as possible with your back straight as you pull your left knee into your chest and feel the stretch in your left glute.

4. Hold the stretch, then repeat on the opposite side.

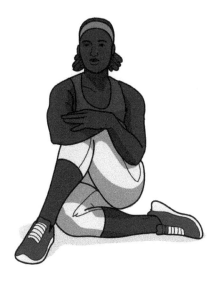

SEATED TOE TOUCH

This stretch is important because it targets your hamstrings.

1. Sit on the ground with your feet out in front of you, legs straight, toes up.

2. Reach both arms straight in front of you and attempt to touch your toes. If you cannot reach your toes, then try for your ankles or shins.

3. Keep your knees as straight as possible and flex your toes toward your shins to maximize the stretch in your hamstrings.

4. Hold the stretch.

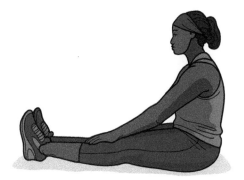

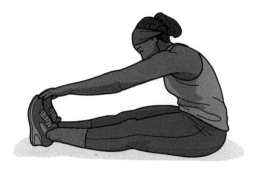

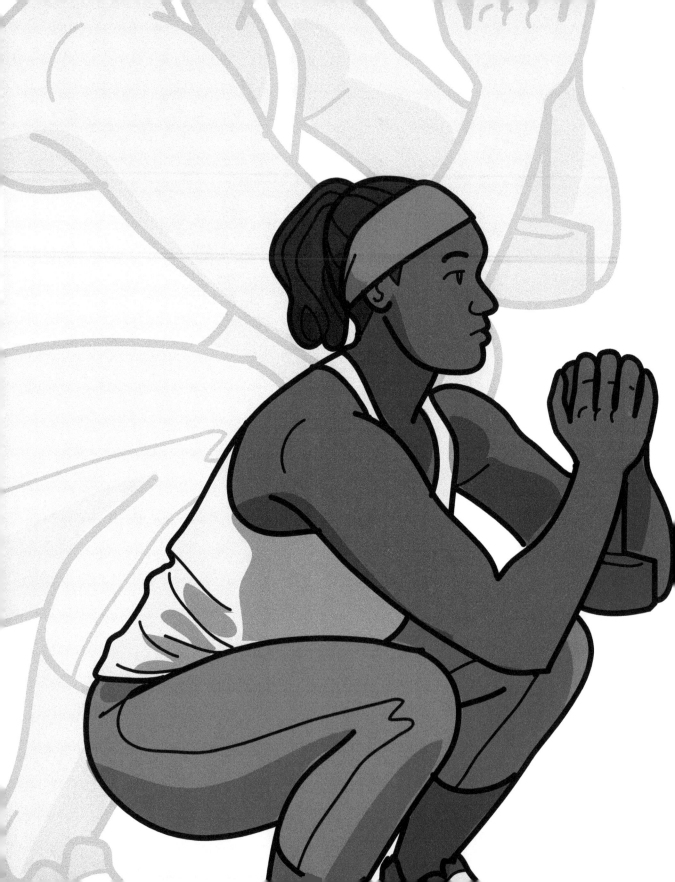

4. QUADRICEPS AND CALVES

The term "quads" is short for the group of muscles in the front of the thigh, collectively known as the quadriceps. This muscle group includes the rectus femoris, vastus medialis, vastus lateralis, and vastus intermedius. The main job of the quads is to straighten or extend the knee. The rectus femoris is a unique muscle because it crosses two joints: the knee and the hip. The other muscle groups in the quads only cross the knee joint. So, the rectus femoris also assists in flexing the hip. Together these muscle groups help you perform activities such as walking, running, jumping, and sitting. This muscle group tends to hold a lot of tension for people who sit for the majority of their days. The reason for this is that when you sit, your quadriceps are in constant contraction, and the constant contraction pulls your pelvic bone forward, which also results in lower back pain. It's a good idea to warm up the quads before engaging in explosive activities like running, jumping, and biking. And if you sit quite a bit throughout your day, it's important to stretch your quadriceps often.

The calves are the muscles in the back of the lower leg. These muscles include the gastrocnemius and soleus. Together they are responsible for pointing and flexing the foot, along with turning the foot inward and outward. The calves are constantly working to maintain your balance and posture while standing or walking; therefore, they're often tight and should be stretched regularly to relieve tension. They're especially active during explosive activities such as running and jumping. The calves are also subject to excess strain if you wear shoes with a heel often, so it is also recommended to stretch and foam roll your calves after wearing heels as an extra self-care practice.

Before You Lift:

Remember to keep your core engaged while executing the movements in this chapter. You can also perform each of these movements in front of a mirror, or record yourself, to double-check your form.

BUTT KICKER

This is a great dynamic warm-up that stretches the quads by forcing them to relax as a result of explosively using the hamstring muscles to flex the knees. This is based on the principle of reciprocal inhibition, which means that one muscle group can't be active while the opposite or opposing muscle group is in use.

1. Stand with your feet hip-width apart and place your hands, palms facing out, on your bottom.

2. Kick one foot up so that your heel smacks the palm of your hand slightly. Then return the foot to the ground and repeat on the opposite side.

3. The motion can be done either jogging in place or while moving forward.

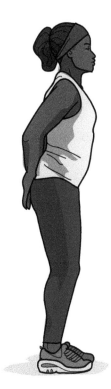

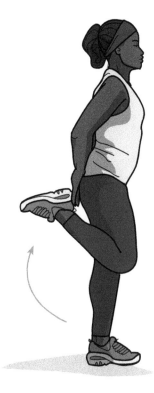

GOBLET SQUAT

ADDITIONAL MUSCLES WORKED: *Core, Glutes, Hamstrings*

Goblet Squats are a great way to perfect your squat form. The counterbalance of front-loaded weight keeps your body from shifting too far forward when you squat. This is because the weight forces your hips to sit back. Think of this motion as sitting down and standing up like you would if you were to sit on a chair—that will help you understand what the movement should feel like.

1. Stand with your feet hip-width apart and toes facing forward, holding a dumbbell with both hands in front of your chest.

2. Push your hips back and imagine yourself sitting down into a chair as you bend at the knees and lower yourself down into a squat position.

3. Stop at the bottom of your squat when your knees and hips form a 90-degree angle.

4. When you're ready to return to standing, press down through your feet and drive up out of the floor to stand, squeezing your glutes at the top.

Lift Safely: Keep your back straight and chest high, and your weight evenly distributed in the middle of your feet throughout the movement. Keep your knees tracking in the same direction as your toes but make sure they stay behind your toes. This is to protect your knees and prevent injury or pain. It also ensures that you are engaging your glutes properly. You can play around with making your stance wider or narrower, or try turning your feet out slightly. Find whatever foot position is optimal for your body type so that you can squat without your spine rounding at the bottom. If you start to feel any discomfort in your back, reduce your range of motion and do not squat as low.

Make It Easier: Put a chair behind you to sit on as you get used to the squatting pattern. You should only feel this exercise in your legs, and in your arms from holding the weight. If you feel any discomfort in your lower back, put the weight down and work on squatting with just body weight.

Home Workout Hack: You can use any item that you have at home as a makeshift weight, including a purse, your baby, a gallon of water, a backpack, a garden pot, heavy books, pet food—get creative!

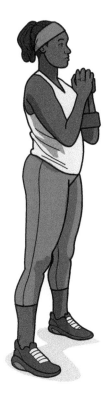

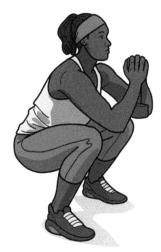

FORWARD LUNGE

ADDITIONAL MUSCLES WORKED: *Glutes, Hamstrings*

This exercise is a functional way to work your quads and calves because it is a similar movement pattern to walking. Lunges also help work your legs unilaterally (one leg at a time). Building strength unilaterally will help your bilateral exercises (squats and Deadlifts) become stronger.

1. Stand with your feet hip-width apart and toes facing forward. Hold dumbbells in both hands down by your sides with your back straight and shoulder blades squeezed together. If using a barbell, place it across your upper back along your shoulders.

2. Take a large step forward and bend both legs to 90-degree angles. Your back knee should hover just above the ground.

3. Drive out of your front heel to step back and return to the starting position. Repeat on the opposite side.

Lift Safely: Make sure your front knee stays behind your front toes as you lunge forward. Your front knee should track in the same line as your ankle and foot. Keep your back straight and chest high as you perform the movement.

Make It Easier: Do your lunges in place and without weight to learn the movement pattern. You can also put your hand against a wall or hold a stick for balance as you learn the movement.

Make It Harder: Perform walking lunges by stepping forward instead of returning to the starting position. To make it even harder, walk continuously without resetting in the middle of the movement by bringing your back leg straight through into another Forward Lunge.

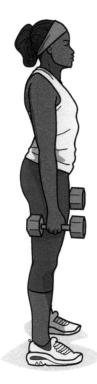

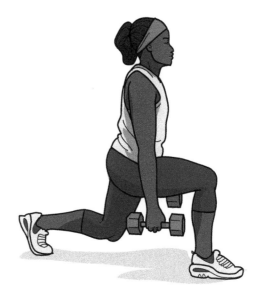

LATERAL LUNGE

ADDITIONAL MUSCLES WORKED: *Glutes, Hamstrings*

It is important to perform exercises in various planes of motion to mimic real-life movements. This exercise is similar to the Forward Lunge, but because it is in the frontal plane (moving side to side), it allows for different muscle activation. You will work more of your outer glute muscles and inner thighs.

1. Stand with your feet hip-width apart and your toes facing forward. Hold dumbbells at your sides in both hands with your back straight and shoulder blades squeezed together. If using a barbell, place it across your upper back along your shoulders.

2. Without turning your body, take a step out to your right and plant your right foot, toes facing forward. Bend your right knee to a 90-degree angle as you lower your hips back and down like you're sitting in a chair. Keep your left leg straight and left toes pointed forward as you do this.

3. Push off the floor with the right foot, putting the weight in your mid foot, and return to the starting position.

4. Repeat on the left side.

Lift Safely: Keep your back flat and chest high as you perform this exercise. Keep your knee behind your toes and tracking over your ankle as you lunge. Your foot should be straight or slightly turned out when you step to the side, and your shoulders square. (Avoid bending your spine in the direction that you're lunging.) You want to keep your hips, knees, and ankles in alignment throughout the movement.

Make It Easier: Perform the exercise with no weights. You may also use a stick or wall to help balance yourself as you learn the movement. Adjusting the depth of your lunge so that you are not lunging as low will make the movement easier as well.

Make It Harder: Perform walking Lateral Lunges instead of staying in place. You can also increase the weight to progress this movement.

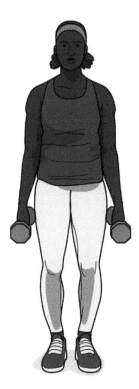

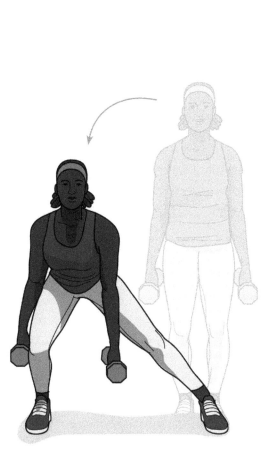

BULGARIAN SPLIT SQUAT

ADDITIONAL MUSCLES WORKED: *Glutes, Hamstrings*

This exercise is just a fancy way of saying that the movement is an in-place, elevated lunge. (The name originated from the Bulgarian weightlifting system.) The elevation requires more balance, which is a great way to work your calves a little more. It also helps develop more strength in each leg independently to help keep your legs balanced in muscle and strength.

1. Stand in front of a chair or box with your feet hip-width apart and facing forward. Place a barbell across your back along your shoulders. If using dumbbells, hold them at your sides or hold one in both hands in front of your chest.

2. Carefully place one foot on the chair behind you so that you are in a split stance. The foot on the chair can be either flat and facedown or the toes can be tucked under, whichever provides you with more stability.

3. Bend your knees and sink into a lunge. Your back knee should hover a few inches from the floor. Both knees should be close to a 90-degree angle at the bottom of the movement.

4. Press into the ground with the heel of your front leg and return to the starting position.

5. Repeat on the opposite side.

Lift Safely: While performing this movement, keep your back straight and chest up. Also, keep your front knee behind your front toes, and your knee tracking in line with your ankle and foot. Make sure the area around you is clear just in case you lose your balance. If you feel discomfort in your knees while performing this movement, adjust your feet and also your depth from the chair. You do not need to go all the way to a 90-degree angle if you don't think you have the stability or strength to do so.

Make It Easier: Choose another chair or surface that's lower to the ground. The higher the chair, the more difficult the exercise will be. To further regress this exercise, perform it without weight.

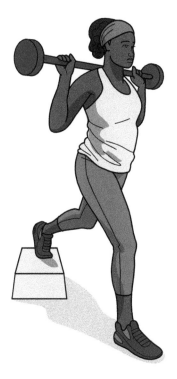

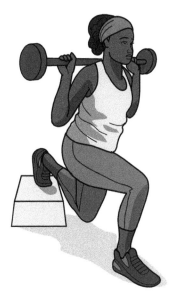

SUITCASE SQUAT

ADDITIONAL MUSCLES WORKED: *Core, Glutes, Hamstrings*

This is another functional movement, as it is similar to how you move when picking up groceries or your suitcases from the floor. It teaches your body how to maneuver a load closer to the ground as opposed to a load closer to your center of mass, like with the Goblet Squats.

1. Stand with your feet hip-width apart and toes facing forward. The dumbbells should be on the ground on either side of your feet.

2. Squat down and grab the dumbbells off the ground. Keep your back straight, chest high, and shoulder blades squeezed together as you squat. Drive out of your feet to return to a standing position, holding the dumbbells.

3. Squat back down to about a 90-degree angle while keeping the dumbbells at the sides of your knees and close to your body. Your weight should be evenly distributed between and in the middle of your feet as you carry the load.

4. Squeeze your glutes and bring your hips forward to return to the upright position, still holding the dumbbells.

5. Repeat this movement for the specified number of reps, then carefully squat down to place the dumbbells back on the ground once you've completed your set.

Lift Safely: Make sure to keep your knees behind your toes and tracking with your ankles as you perform this movement. If you feel discomfort in your lower back, place the weights down and adjust the position of your feet. You may also reduce the depth that you are squatting. Pay attention to your first and last reps. These are when you'll be picking up the dumbbells and putting them back down, and people most often injure themselves doing the first or last rep of a loaded exercise.

Make It Harder: Perform the movement with only one dumbbell. This will force your core to activate more in order to counteract the effects of the dumbbell only weighing down one side of your body.

Home Workout Hack: Practice this at home with your groceries or suitcases the next time you go shopping or travel.

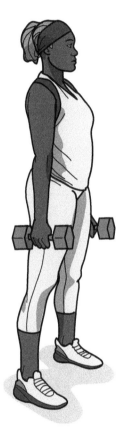

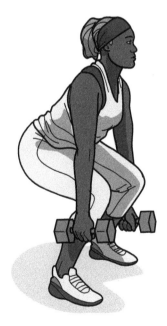

SINGLE-LEG GOBLET SQUAT

ADDITIONAL MUSCLES WORKED: *Biceps, Core, Glutes, Hamstrings*

This movement is a modified pistol squat. It is great for challenging your balance and for unilateral (single side) strength. The regular Goblet Squat works bilateral (both sides) strength, so this a progression of that exercise.

1. Stand in front of a chair or box with your feet hip-width apart. Hold a dumbbell in front of your chest with both hands, or a barbell across your upper back along your shoulders.

2. Raise one foot into the air and carefully lower yourself down to sit in the chair. To raise your leg, you can either lift your foot and bend your knee or lift your entire leg out in front of you without bending your knee. Use whichever method is easier.

3. Keeping the same foot elevated and using your other leg, stand up out of the chair.

4. You may place your foot down on the floor to regain stability before continuing on to the next repetition.

5. Repeat on the other leg.

Lift Safely: Be sure to control your momentum as you squat down to the chair. Don't just flop down on the chair. Keep your knees behind your toes and tracking with your ankle as you squat down and stand up, and keep your foot pointed forward.

Make It Easier: You can choose a taller chair or place a book on the chair to make it easier to stand up. You can also regress this exercise by not using the weight. Additionally, you can stand up with both legs and sit down with one leg until you have the strength to stand up with only one leg.

Make It Harder: You can use a shorter chair to make this more difficult. You can also lose the chair and just do pistol squats while holding the weight.

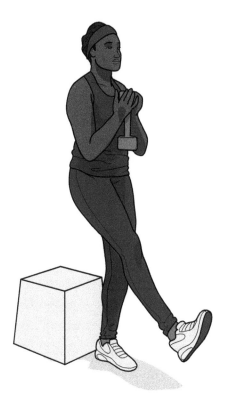

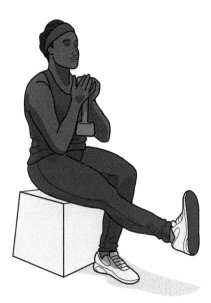

CURTSY LUNGE

ADDITIONAL MUSCLES WORKED: *Glutes, Hamstrings*

This is another exercise that works your muscles in a different plane of motion: the transverse plane. Rotational movements are done in the transverse plane and include basically any twisting action. This movement also helps strengthen your vastus medialis oblique, which is a thigh muscle that is often underactive. Strengthening this muscle can help reduce the risk of knee injuries in females, especially female athletes who play sports that involve cutting movements, like soccer, basketball, and tennis.

1. Stand with your feet hip-width apart and toes facing forward. Hold dumbbells at your sides with your shoulder blades squeezed together and neck relaxed. If using a barbell, hold it across your upper back along your shoulders.

2. Take one foot and cross it behind the other foot as you lower yourself down into a lunge. You should feel like you're curtsying to the Queen of England.

3. Aim to have both of your knees at a 90-degree angle with your hips at the bottom of your lunge.

4. Return your back foot to the starting position. Repeat on the opposite side.

Lift Safely: Keep your hips, knees, and ankles in alignment throughout the movement. Your front knee should track with your ankle and toes as you lunge—without extending beyond your toes—and your shoulders should remain square and facing forward. There should be no rotation in your back or hips when performing this movement. Keep your back straight the entire time.

Make It Easier: Keep your feet in a fixed curtsy position and practice the lunge in place to learn the movement. You may also hold on to something to help bear some of your weight as you learn the movement.

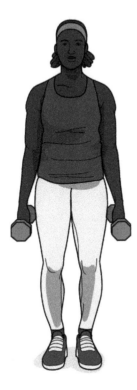

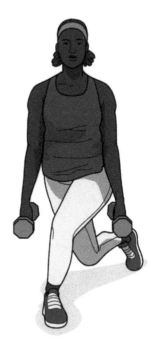

STANDING CALF STRETCH

Use this standing stretch to release the tension in your calves as you cool down after performing the previous exercises so that you avoid cramping post-workout.

1. Stand with one foot flat on the ground, in front of the other, and flex your front toes toward the sky.

2. Bend forward and grab your front toes. Keep your knees as straight as possible.

3. Pull your toes toward your shin until you feel a stretch in your calf. You may also feel a stretch in your hamstrings, which is fine.

4. Repeat on the opposite side.

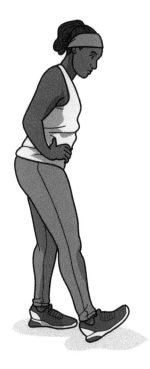

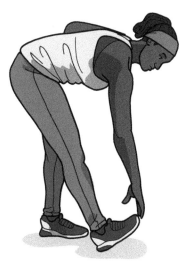

STANDING QUAD STRETCH

The quads are a large group of muscles that tend to be very active in women. It is important to stretch them after a leg workout. This stretch is an easy one that you can do anywhere.

1. Stand with your feet hip-width apart.

2. Bend your right knee so that your right leg lifts from the ground and moves toward your butt.

3. Grab your right ankle with your right hand. Pull your foot toward your butt until you feel a stretch in your right quad.

4. Carefully release the foot and return it to the floor.

5. Repeat on the opposite side.

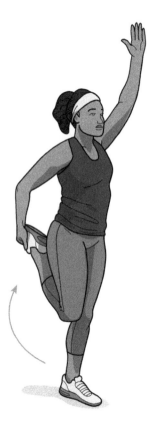

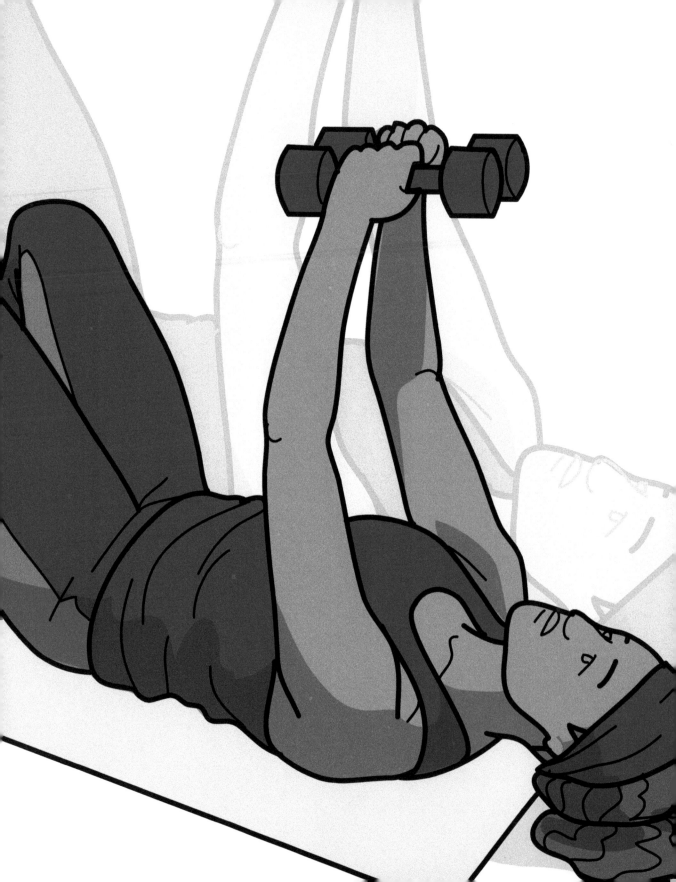

5. CHEST

The chest is composed of a layer of muscles that start in your décolletage and extend under your breasts. This large muscle group is made up of the pectoralis major and pectoralis minor. This is why you may have heard people refer to their chests as their "pecs."

Working your chest muscles is a great way to give yourself a natural breast lift if you have an aesthetic-based goal. Some women worry that doing chest exercises will make their chest smaller by turning their breast tissue into muscle–this is not the case. If a reduction in your breast size occurs, it's due to the weight loss that you're experiencing as a result of general weightlifting. The same effect could happen if you lost weight doing only cardio. Everyone has different genetics, which means you can't control where and when your body will lose weight. You can't spot train, meaning you can't work a particular muscle group hoping to lose fat in that specific area. I hope that this helps ease any reservations that you may have about training your chest. The benefits of building strength outweigh the risk of dropping a cup size due to general weight loss. As a side note, if you've had a breast augmentation, then you may need to take special precautions when working your chest. You may need to use lighter weights and/or reduce your range of motion. This is because of the scar tissue that you may have as a result of the augmentation. It's also so that the appearance of your breasts is not affected due to the implants shifting. Consult your surgeon on recommendations and best practices.

Before You Lift:

Remember to keep your core engaged while executing the movements in this chapter. You can also perform each of these movements in front of a mirror, or record yourself, to double-check your form.

SCAPTION PLANK

Scaptions are a great way to get your shoulder blades moving better. The muscles that surround your shoulder blades play an essential role in pushing and pulling exercises—specifically in relationship to chest movements—so you want to make sure they are sufficiently warmed.

1. Begin with your arms extended, in a push-up position, with your wrists stacked under your shoulders and toes on the floor hip-width apart. Create one long line from your head to your heels.

2. With your elbows locked and arms straight, pull your shoulder blades toward your spine (retraction).

3. In the same position, push your shoulder blades away from each other, away from your spine and closer to your shoulders (protraction). Repeat the retracting and protracting movements; practice pushing your shoulders toward and then away from each other.

4. Try to get as much movement as possible with your shoulder blades without moving your neck. You may also perform this movement standing up, with your hands against a wall.

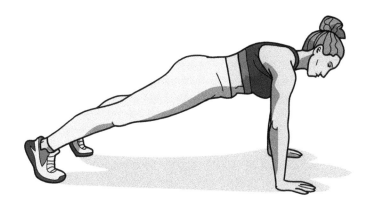

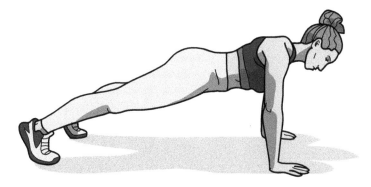

DUMBBELL FLOOR PRESS

ADDITIONAL MUSCLES WORKED: *Triceps*

This is a fundamental pushing movement. It uses both of your pectoral muscles, and by using the dumbbells as opposed to a barbell, you can work on building strength in each arm independently. This movement is also recommended over a traditional bench press (on a flat bench with a barbell) if you've had a breast augmentation.

1. Lie on your back on the floor with your knees bent and feet flat on the ground hip-width apart. Have the dumbbells by your sides near your hands so that you can reach them easily.

2. With your arms straight and elbows locked, lift the weights above you so that they are directly above your chest. You want your thumbs to be facing each other so that your palms are facing out and the dumbbells are horizontal to each other.

3. Lower the dumbbells down to your chest simultaneously by bending your elbows to 90 degrees, taking them wide and away from each other. Stop once your elbows touch the ground.

4. Press the weights back up by bringing your elbows in toward each other to return to the starting position.

Lift Safely: Keep your lower back flat against the floor, rib cage down, as you perform this exercise. Avoid arching your back—this will help keep your core activated. Don't lock your elbows at the top of the movement.

Make It Harder: You can make this exercise a little harder by lifting both feet into the air so that you're in an upside-down tabletop position with your knees over your hips and your calves parallel to the ground. This will require more core stability. You can also only press one dumbbell at a time. This will require more stabilization to counteract the rotational force produced by having an imbalance in weight distribution.

Home Workout Hack: If you are looking to strengthen your chest without the use of weights, then do push-ups. You can make push-ups easier by doing them on your knees or by putting your hands on an elevated surface like a bench or counter top.

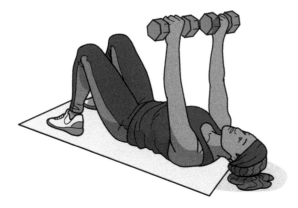

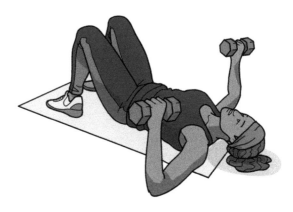

DUMBBELL CHEST FLY

ADDITIONAL MUSCLES WORKED: *Triceps*

This exercise works the chest slightly different from the Dumbbell Floor Press. It will strengthen the areas in your chest that can help your breasts appear closer together. Building strength is the focus of this exercise, but the extra aesthetic benefits are nice to note. It's also worth noting that this will be a more friendly chest exercise than the Barbell Floor Press if you've had breast augmentation.

1. Lie on your back with your knees bent, feet flat on the floor, hip-width apart. The dumbbells should be at your sides and close to your hands so that you can easily pick them up.

2. Pick up the weights with arms extended, and bring them above your chest, palms facing each other with your thumbs pointing toward your face.

3. Open your arms, with elbows slightly bent, as if you were getting ready to hug a tree or grab a giant beach ball.

4. Lower the weights toward the floor and stop when your elbows are at chest height. This will be just a few inches above the ground. Do not let the weights rest on the ground.

5. Return your arms to the starting position by squeezing your elbows toward each other.

Lift Safely: Keep your lower back flat against the floor as you perform this exercise. Don't arch your back—this will help keep your core activated. Don't overextend your arms on the way down. Stop when you feel a comfortable stretch in your chest. Keep the weights just in front of your chest as you perform this movement. They shouldn't be up by your neck/head, and they shouldn't be down by your belly button.

Make It Harder: Perform the exercise with your feet off the ground, knees over hips and calves parallel to the floor, to require more core engagement. You can also use only one dumbbell to make it harder or alternate sides instead of moving the weights at the same time.

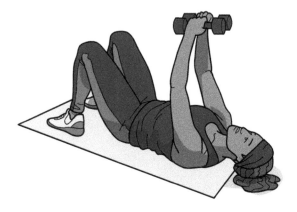

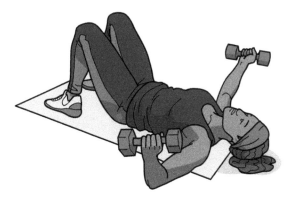

WIDE-GRIP BARBELL CHEST PRESS

ADDITIONAL MUSCLES WORKED: *Triceps*

The use of a wide grip in this press will target a different part of the chest muscles than the other chest exercises mentioned in this chapter. It will help keep your muscles balanced and at an optimal strength level for pressing.

1. Lie on your back with your knees bent, feet flat on the floor, hip-width apart. You should have your barbell in your hands as you lie down.

2. Grip the barbell directly above your chest with hands wide; think about bringing your pinkies as close to the weighted ends of the barbell as you can.

3. Lower the bar down toward your chest, keeping it centered above the middle of your chest. Stop once your elbows touch the floor.

4. Press the bar back up by squeezing your elbows in toward each other.

Lift Safely: Keep your lower back flat against the ground as you press the weight. Don't arch your back. Keep your wrists straight and rib cage down as you press. Once you've finished the exercise, sit up carefully with the bar by engaging your core and rolling up to a seated position facing forward. Don't attempt to push the bar off behind you or to the side of you. If you have a spotter around to assist in taking the barbell away from you, that would be ideal. You may need to use lighter weight or avoid this movement if you've had breast augmentation.

Make It Harder: Perform the exercise with your feet off the ground, knees over hips and calves parallel to the floor, to require more core engagement.

Home Workout Hack: If you don't have a barbell, then perform push-ups with your hands wider than shoulder-width apart. Your hands should be placed 2 inches outside of the shoulder joint. You can also do an elevated wide push-up by putting your hands on a bench or counter top. This is also a great alternative if you're looking to build strength in your chest and you've had breast augmentation.

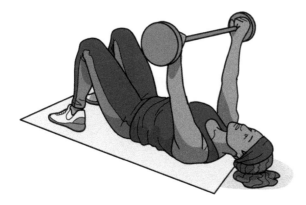

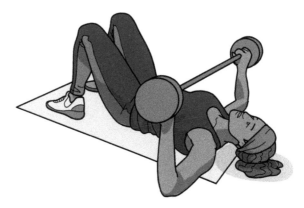

WALL STRETCH

The chest muscles tend to be very tight from daily activities like driving, typing, and texting. Exercising this muscle group leads to even more tightness, so it's very important to stretch post-workout to help return the muscle to its original length. It's also a good idea to perform this Wall Stretch after a long period of sitting at a computer or behind the wheel of your car. A tight chest can lead to shoulder impingements and lack of shoulder mobility.

1. Stand in a doorway with the doorframe on your right side. Place your left foot slightly in front of you and your right foot slightly behind.

2. Place your right hand on the doorframe so that your elbow is at a 90-degree angle directly in line with your shoulder.

3. Press your body forward while you simultaneously press your arm into the doorframe, until you feel a stretch in your chest. Avoid arching your back as you do this.

4. Repeat on the opposite side.

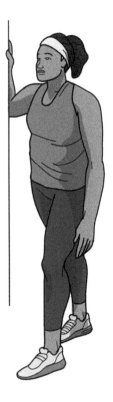

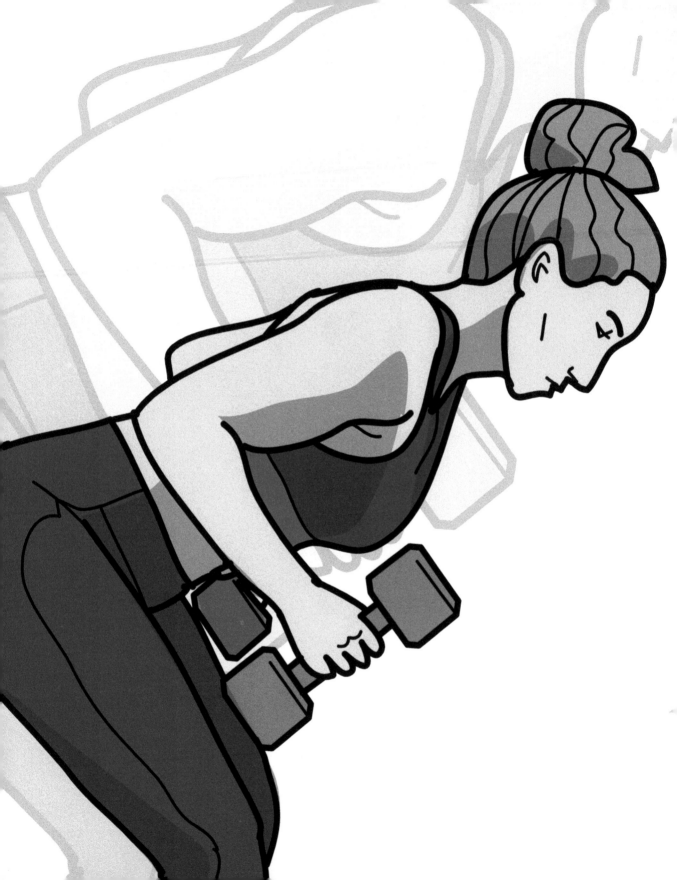

6. UPPER BACK

The upper back is composed of a few large muscle groups, including the trapezius and rhomboids. The trapezius muscles, or "traps," run from the base of your skull all the way to the middle of your spine. You have upper, middle, and lower traps, which are responsible for different actions, such as elevating and depressing your shoulders, and rotating and retracting the shoulder blades. The traps also assist in turning the neck and head. If you spend a lot of time sitting at a desk, then you may often experience tension in your upper traps.

The rhomboids are mainly responsible for squeezing your shoulder blades together. Strengthening your rhomboids can greatly help improve your posture. The rhomboids perform the opposite motion of your chest (pulling); therefore, it's important to work the rhomboids to counteract all of the pushing movements that you do throughout the day.

Another important group of muscles in your upper back are the muscles that stabilize and move your scapula (shoulder blade). These muscles are collectively known as your rotator cuff muscles. They help stabilize your shoulders and also allow movements such as elevation, depression, retraction, protraction, upward rotation, and downward rotation. Basically, all of the fun movements that you can do with your shoulders are controlled by your shoulder blades and rotator cuff muscles.

Before You Lift:

Remember to keep your core engaged while executing the movements in this chapter. You can also perform each of these movements in front of a mirror, or record yourself, to double-check your form.

T-SPINE ROTATION

It is really important to warm up and stretch your upper back to help with mobility of your thoracic spine, or T-spine, which is the middle of your back. Oftentimes the middle of your back can lose mobility due to sitting too long or as a result of other muscular imbalances. Performing this stretch will help you regain some mobility, which will ultimately help your weightlifting be more effective.

1. Lie on your side. Reach both arms straight out in front of your chest with your palms pressed together.

2. Straighten your bottom leg and bend the knee of your top leg so that it's at a 90-degree angle.

3. Slowly take your top hand and open it to the opposite side of the floor while twisting through your mid back and head so that your eyes are following your hand.

4. Your arms should be straight at 180 degrees at the end of the stretch, with your head facing the opposite direction and your top knee still bent.

5. Slowly return to the starting position and repeat on the opposite side.

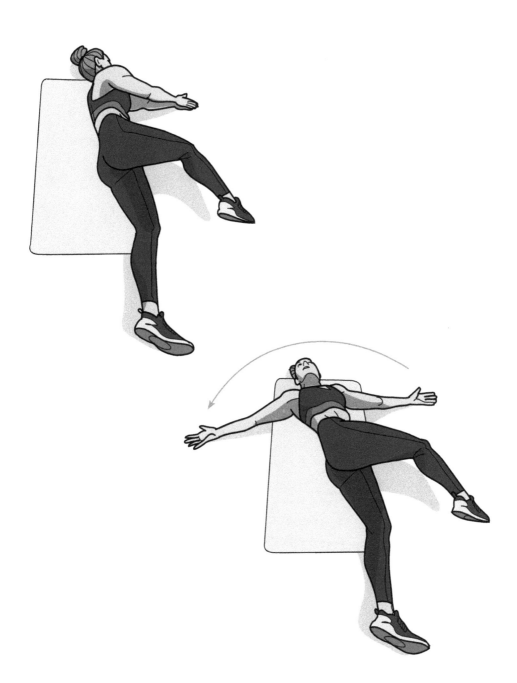

BENT-OVER ROW

ADDITIONAL MUSCLES WORKED: *Biceps, Core*

This movement specifically targets the rhomboids and assists in creating better posture. It's also a great exercise to help reinforce the deadlifting movement pattern. A strong Bent-Over Row will help improve the strength level of your other back exercises since you are engaging your middle and lower back muscles.

1. Stand tall with your feet under your hips, holding dumbbells at your sides or a barbell in front of you, hands gripping the bar just outside your thighs.

2. Hinge at the hips and lower your chest down toward the ground. You want to keep your back as straight and flat as possible as you do this. The weights should now be parallel to your chest with your palms facing each other.

3. Bend both elbows simultaneously and row the weights up until they reach your ribs. Squeeze your shoulder blades together at the top of this movement.

4. Slowly return the weights to the starting position by straightening your elbows.

5. Remain in the bent-over position until all repetitions are completed, then return to the starting upright position.

Lift Safely: Keep your back completely flat throughout the movement. Don't round the middle of your spine or arch your lower back while performing the movement. Engage the muscles in the middle of your back as opposed to using your upper traps. Do this by drawing your shoulder blades down and squeezing them together. Keep your shoulders as relaxed as possible and your neck in a neutral position.

Make It Easier: If it's too hard to hold the bent position, you can hold one dumbbell in one hand and use the other hand to support your weight on a chair. Use the chair to help stabilize your core and to find the correct neutral spine position needed for this exercise.

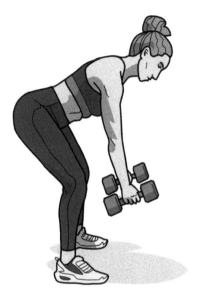

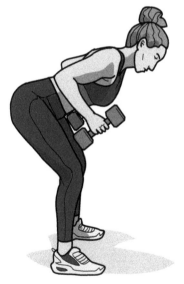

REVERSE FLY

ADDITIONAL MUSCLES WORKED: *Core, Shoulders*

This exercise is really good for working some of the smaller muscles in and around your rotator cuff muscles. It's also a great way to improve your posture and overall strength. This movement is similar to Bent-Over Rows but is much more difficult due to the use of smaller muscle groups.

1. Stand with your feet hip-width apart holding dumbbells by your sides.

2. Hinge at the hips and keep your back straight and flat as you lower your chest toward the floor. The weights should now be parallel to your chest with your palms facing each other.

3. Keeping your arms straight and elbows slightly bent, extend both arms straight out to your sides to form a long line. Picture yourself as a bird extending your wings to fly and squeeze your shoulder blades together at the top of the motion.

4. Return the weights to the center of your body just in front of your chest.

Lift Safely: Lift the weights in a slow, controlled motion. Avoid jerking your neck forward or raising your chest to try to use momentum to get the weights up. Don't overextend your arms. Perform the movement within a comfortable range of motion. Avoid arching your lower back.

Home Workout Hack: This is a great exercise to try with a resistance band. Simply hold the opposite ends of the band (as opposed to holding the handles). Pull the band apart like you're trying to rip it into two pieces.

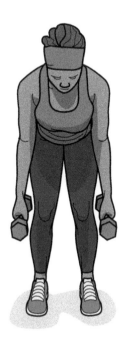

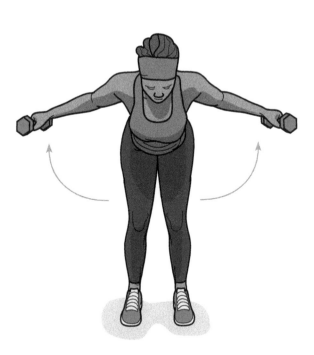

FARMER'S CARRY

ADDITIONAL MUSCLES WORKED: *Core*

This is another exercise designed to help you improve your posture. It's also a very functional exercise as it is similar to movements that you do every week, like carrying grocery bags. Keep this exercise in mind the next time you carry shopping bags or your purse.

1. Stand with your feet hip-width apart and hold dumbbells at your sides.

2. Walk in a straight line for a few steps and then turn around and walk back.

3. As you walk, brace your core and squeeze your shoulder blades together to maintain upright posture. You want to think about having the best posture possible while walking around with your dumbbells. The dumbbells should be heavy enough that you feel your core engaging as you walk, and you should also feel your shoulders depressing slightly.

Lift Safely: Pay close attention to how you pick up and put back down your dumbbells before and after the exercise. Use good squat form when doing this. Avoid bending over and rounding your back when handling the weights.

Make It Harder: Perform the exercise using only one weight; this will require more core engagement and balance. You can also make it harder by walking slower.

Home Workout Hack: A Farmer's Carry can be done with many different items. This exercise is named because farmers often carry the various items on their farms this way. Get creative and see what items in your home you can Farmer Carry, for example, buckets, gardening supplies, backpacks, and luggage.

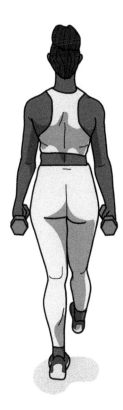

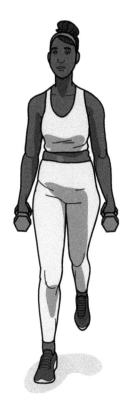

CAT-COW

Cat-Cow is another good movement to do to increase your thoracic mobility. It is particularly good for people who have forward shoulders and/or a rounded spine. Cat-Cow helps you learn how to get your spine back to a neutral position for weightlifting and other movements.

1. Start in a quadruped position (on your hands and knees with your palms flat on the ground) with your knees directly under your hips, toes on the ground, and wrists under your shoulders.

2. Drop your head down, round your back, and tuck your hips under to form a shape like a cat.

3. Lift your head up and arch your lower back by pressing your stomach toward the floor to form a shape similar to a cow.

4. Repeat the movement, flowing fluidly between cat and then cow.

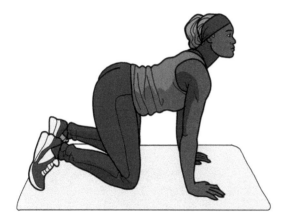

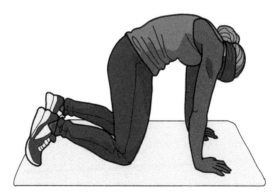

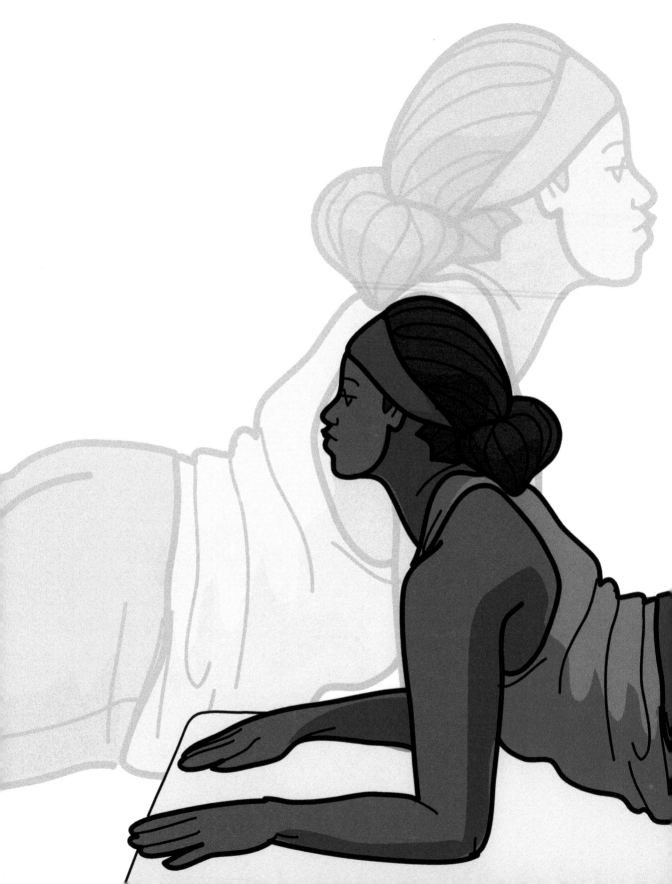

7. LOWER BACK

Many people suffer from lower back pain. This is sometimes the result of having weak muscles in the lower back or, more often than not, a weak core. To avoid lower back pain, it's important to strengthen your lower back by doing functional exercises that build stability. If we take a look at the "joint-by-joint approach" (a theory that the body is made up of alternating stable and mobile joints), we will see that the lower back should be a stable joint. If you suffer a lack of mobility in your hip joints or thoracic spine (T-spine), then your lower back will sacrifice stability for extra mobility to compensate for your lack of hip and T-spine mobility. As you can see, sometimes it is not a lack of strength that is the issue, but rather a lack of stability.

The explanation above should help ease any hesitation or concern that you may have about weightlifting for your lower back. Everything in this chapter is meant to strengthen your core and stabilize your lower back. Functional strength is the key to avoiding general lower back pain.

Before You Lift:

Remember to keep your core engaged while executing the movements in this chapter. You can also perform each of these movements in front of a mirror, or record yourself, to double-check your form.

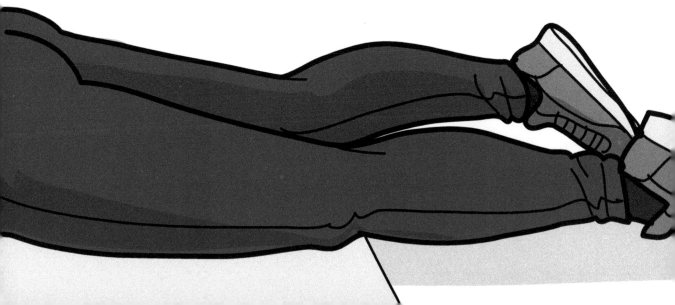

T-SPINE ROTATION

The reason this exercise is included again as a warm-up for your lower back is that a mobile T-spine will help your lower back stabilize while you perform the exercises in this chapter. Remember, your body works together as one big kinetic chain. Every muscle or joint helps another achieve a desired movement.

1. Lie on your side. Reach both arms straight out in front of your chest with your palms pressed together.

2. Straighten your bottom leg and bend the knee of your top leg so that it's at a 90-degree angle.

3. Slowly take your top hand and open it to the opposite side of the floor while twisting through your mid back and head so that your eyes are following your hand.

4. Your arms should be straight at 180 degrees at the end of the stretch, with your head facing the opposite direction and your top knee still bent.

5. Slowly return to the starting position and repeat on the opposite side.

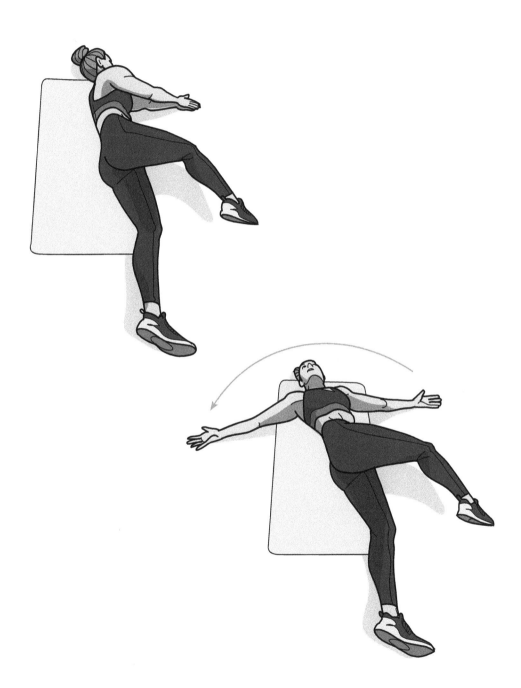

DUMBBELL BIRD-DOG

ADDITIONAL MUSCLES WORKED: *Core, Glutes, Shoulders*

A proper Bird-Dog is a very effective core stabilizer. It teaches your lower back how to stay stable while you move your arms and legs. This is an essential skill to have when performing most weightlifting exercises.

1. Begin in a quadruped position (on your hands and knees) on the floor with a dumbbell in front of you. Have your hips stacked over your knees and your shoulders stacked over your wrists.

2. Stabilize your back in a neutral position by keeping your lower back from arching and your mid back from rounding. Your neck should also be neutral; do not bend or extend it. Imagine a pole on your back that you want to maintain contact with your head, mid back, and tailbone.

3. Grab the dumbbell in front of you and extend your arm straight forward with your palm facing inward. At the same time, extend your opposite leg behind you. Keep your feet flexed and act like you're trying to kick the wall behind you with your heel that's elevated.

4. Return your hand and foot to the ground at the same time, while still keeping your spine neutral.

5. Repeat on the opposite side.

Lift Safely: Work on finding that neutral position with your spine and maintaining it throughout the movement. A neutral spine is the natural curvature that your spine should have at rest. There should not be any excessive flexion or extension happening.

Make It Easier: Perform this movement without the weight or reduce the range of motion.

Make It Harder: If you really want to work your entire back and build strength, perform pull-ups. You can do them at home by attaching a pull-up bar to your doorframe. You can also do assisted pull-ups at home by purchasing a chin-up max to attach to your pull-up bar. Most gyms have an assisted pull-up machine as well if you're unable to do pull-ups.

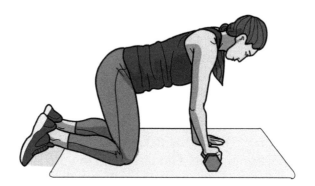

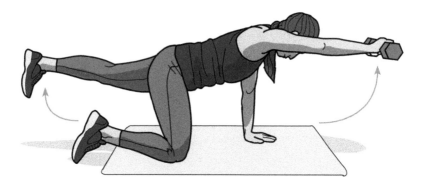

GOOD MORNING

ADDITIONAL MUSCLES WORKED: *Glutes, Hamstrings*

This exercise helps strengthen the erector muscles in the lower back. It is recommended for people who have already mastered the Deadlift hip-hinge pattern and don't currently have a lower back injury.

1. Stand with your feet hip-width apart and toes facing forward.

2. Hold a dumbbell with two hands at your chest and close to your body.

3. Hinge at your hips and keep your back flat as you bend and lower your chest toward the floor. Stop once you feel a good stretch in your hamstrings.

4. Squeeze your glutes to return to the upright position.

Lift Safely: Keep your back flat as you perform this movement. Do not bend your spine or arch your back. Go only as far down as your hip mobility allows. If you start to feel your lower back round at all, stop at that point and return upright.

Make It Easier: Perform this movement without the weight.

Make It Harder: You can hold a barbell on your upper back to load yourself with more weight. Also, having the load on your back as opposed to the front of your body increases the difficulty of the exercise.

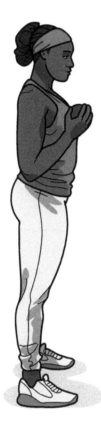

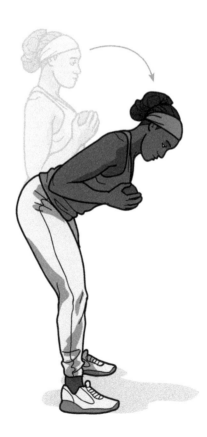

CHILD'S POSE

This movement is really good for stretching the upper and lower back, as well as stretching the shoulders. It's also a relaxing position for most people and can help increase range of motion in the hips and ankles. Better mobility in all of these joints can help relieve pressure in your lower back.

1. Get in a quadruped position (on your hands and knees) on the ground, with your hands under your shoulders and your knees under your hips, or wider if comfortable.

2. Untuck your toes and lay them flat and facedown on the ground. Extend both arms forward as you rock your hips back toward your heels.

3. Try to flatten out your back as much as possible as you reach your arms forward and your hips back. Your chest should be parallel to the floor and your forehead down when you hit the end range of the stretch.

4. When you feel sufficiently stretched, return to the quadruped position by driving your hips and shoulders forward.

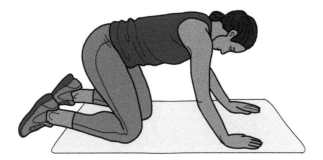

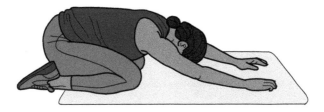

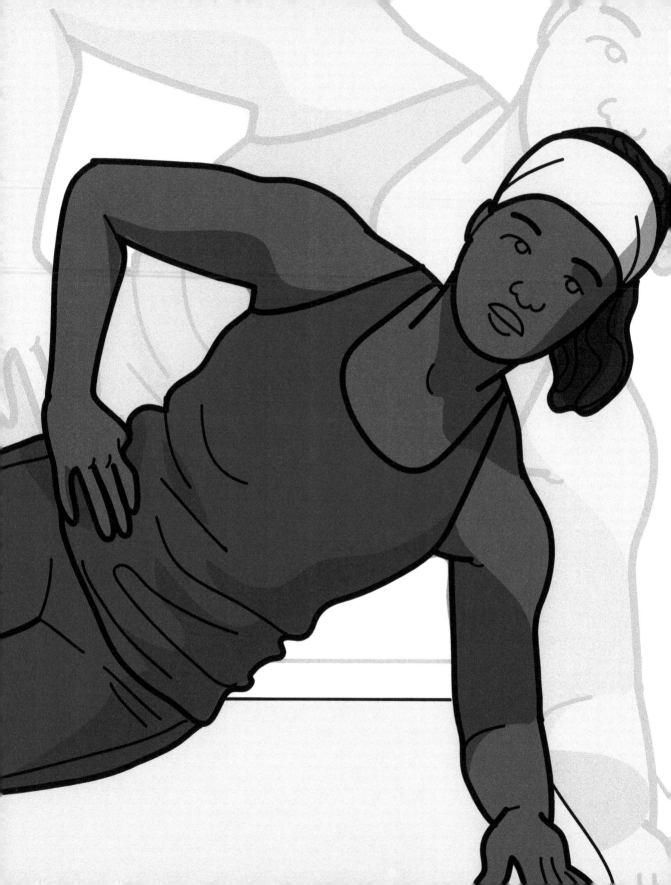

8. ABDOMINALS AND OBLIQUES

Abs are the muscle group that everyone wants to appear flat and struggles to keep when they get them. The muscle group most people think of when you say "abs" is called the rectus abdominis, also commonly referred to as the "six-pack." Genetics determine how the fascia of your rectus abdominis is shaped and how it appears on your body. This is why some people have square abs and others have long abs. This is also why some people have a natural six-pack, while others have an eight- or four-pack. Everyone has abs, but most people can't see their abs because they're hiding behind a layer of fat. No matter how much you work your abs, you cannot change how many you see and their shape. If you want to be able to see your rectus abdominis, then you will need to work on your diet and decrease your body fat.

Your abdominal muscles are divided into four groups. Starting from the outside layer going in, they are the external obliques, rectus abdominis, internal obliques, and the transverse abdominis. The transverse abdominis is the deepest of the abdominal muscles and extends between the ribs and the hips and wraps the core from front to back. This is your most important ab muscle! It's in charge of supporting your organs, assisting with forceful exhalation, and stabilizing your lower back and pelvic floor. This muscle works together with your other abdominals and pelvic floor muscles to stabilize your lower back. Strengthening this muscle will greatly increase your core stability and your ability to lift heavier weights.

Your external and internal obliques (located on the sides of your trunk) assist you with twisting and flexing from side to side. It's important to strengthen these muscle groups if you participate in day-to-day activities that require rotation.

Before You Lift:

Remember to engage your core by drawing your belly button into your spine to target deep core muscles. When you exhale, act like you're trying to fog up a window or blow up a balloon. Keep this feeling in mind while you complete these exercises because you should feel your core engaged at all times. If you start to feel discomfort in your hip flexors or lower back, stop the exercise, reset, and focus on engaging your core.

PLANK

This is an amazing exercise to activate your transverse abdominis along with your other deep core muscles. In doing so, your core will be much stronger and able to support you more effectively as you perform other exercises. In general, Plank is a great warm-up to do before training any muscle group since your core should be engaged with all lifts.

1. Begin in a prone position (on your stomach) facing the floor, with your elbows directly under your shoulders and knees and toes on the ground. Your feet should be about hip-width apart.

2. Slowly lift your knees off the ground and hold this position, keeping your hips level with your shoulders.

3. Imagine you have a pole on your back that you're trying to keep in contact with your head, mid back, and butt. You don't want to have your lower back arched.

4. Actively squeeze your glutes and forcefully press down into the ground with your forearms. You can also pretend like you're trying to drag your elbows to your rib cage without moving them.

5. Release your knees to the ground once you've completed the exercise.

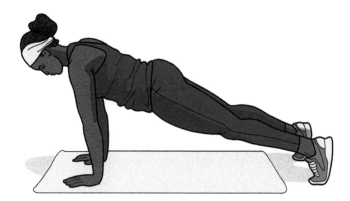

SIDE BRIDGE

ADDITIONAL MUSCLES WORKED: *Glutes, Shoulders*

This exercise helps strengthen your obliques and deep core muscles. The movement pattern also helps reinforce the hip extension needed for squats and Deadlifts. The motion of lifting your hips off the ground while having your top foot in front mimics the hip extension seen in power movements.

1. Lie on your side with your legs straight and your top foot in front of your bottom foot. Make sure that you're lying on your forearm with your elbow stacked directly below your shoulder.

2. Slowly lift your hips off the ground and hold the elevated position, driving your top hip toward the ceiling.

3. You can either keep your opposite hand on your side or raise it into the air, parallel with your shoulder.

Make It Easier: You can keep your bottom knee on the ground. Extend your top leg and bend your bottom knee to bring your bottom foot behind you.

Make It Harder: Once in the full Side Bridge, you can lift up your top leg and hover, or make it even harder by flexing that knee in toward your chest. Return your foot to the starting position on the ground. Repeat for the desired number of reps or seconds. You can also hold a dumbbell in your top hand to make this a weighted movement.

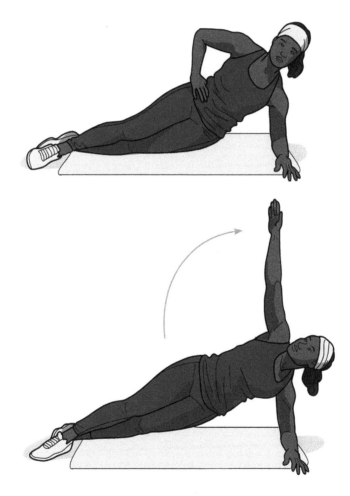

HOLLOW-BODY HOLD

ADDITIONAL MUSCLES WORKED: *Back, Quads*

This is an excellent move to learn how to coordinate your upper and lower halves. It's also a good way to prepare your body for handstands, if that's a goal of yours.

1. Lie flat on your back with your arms extended over your head and legs straight. Keep your feet together and hands facing each other.

2. Slowly raise your shoulder blades off the ground, reaching your hands up and out behind you as you lift your feet off the ground a few inches.

3. Hold this elevated position and think about making your body as long as possible without letting your lower back arch. Keep your lower back pressed into the floor.

4. Return to the starting position.

Lift Safely: Even though you aren't lifting any weight with this exercise, you still want to be conscious of how you are using your body weight. Make sure to keep your neck and shoulders relaxed. Don't thrust your head and neck forward as you raise your shoulder blades off the ground. Also, protect your lower back by making sure there's no space between your back and the ground as you lift your feet off the ground. Be sure to remember to continue breathing during your hold.

Make It Easier: Instead of extending your arms over your head, you can keep your hands down by your sides to modify the hold. As you raise your body to the hold position, reach your arms toward your heels and think about making your body as long as possible.

Make It Harder: Hold a dumbbell with both hands.

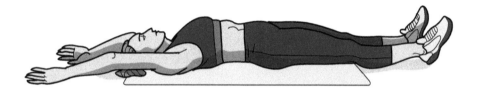

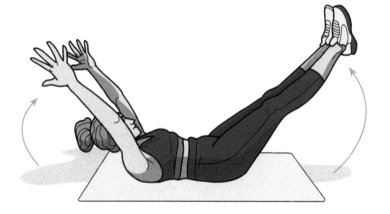

LOWER-LEG LIFT

ADDITIONAL MUSCLES WORKED: *Quads*

This is a challenging ab exercise that allows you to work your abs without flexing your spine. You want to avoid flexing your spine at all costs so that you don't strain your back.

1. Lie on your back with your legs raised to a comfortable height and hands by your sides. Make sure that your lower back is completely flat against the ground.

2. Slowly lower your feet toward the ground and stop when you feel your lower back start to arch. Ideally, you'll be able to build up enough strength to get your feet a few inches from the floor.

3. Engage your abs to pull your legs back up to the starting position.

Lift Safely: Keep your lower back completely flat against the ground throughout the entire movement. You don't want to arch your lower back at all. Keep your head down on the ground with your neck and shoulders as relaxed as possible. If you can't perform this movement without arching your back, then discontinue this exercise and work on strengthening your core with the other exercises mentioned in this chapter.

Make It Easier: Place your hands underneath your butt just where your lower back and tailbone connect. Keep your hands there as you perform the movement. As you gain more core control, you'll be able to remove your hands when performing your leg lifts.

Make It Harder: Hold dumbbells or a barbell above your chest and keep it still as you lift and lower your legs.

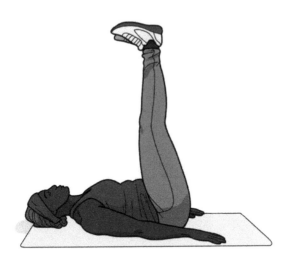

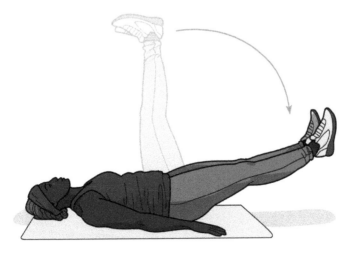

DEAD BUG

ADDITIONAL MUSCLES WORKED: *Quads, Shoulders*

The Dead Bug is a fantastic ab exercise for all fitness levels. It's a safe movement for most people who have back pain and will help strengthen the core to potentially reduce back pain.

1. Lie on your back. Bring your knees up over your hips, your feet and calves parallel to the floor.

2. Extend your arms so that they are straight above your chest.

3. Keep your lower back completely flat on the ground as you extend your left arm back behind your head and extend your right leg straight out in front of you.

4. Return your hand and foot to the starting position and repeat on the opposite side. With this back-and-forth movement of your arms and legs, you should look like a dying bug.

5. Keep your head down on the ground as you perform the movement.

Make It Harder: If you have a foam roller, place it horizontally across the tops of your thighs, holding it in place with your hands. Press the foam roller into your thighs firmly. Now take one hand off the foam roller and extend the hand over your head as you extend the opposite leg. As you are moving the arm and leg, your other arm and leg should still be firmly in contact with the foam roller. Repeat on the opposite side. You may also use a stability ball for this progression, or use dumbbells in each hand to make this a weighted movement.

Home Workout Hack: Here is a trick to learn how to tilt your pelvis so that your lower back remains flat against the ground as you perform various ab exercises like this one: Roll up a towel lengthwise and place it under your lower back. It should be in the small of your back between your butt and rib cage with the ends extending out past your sides. Lift your legs and attempt to smash the towel with your lower back. Now grab the towel and attempt to slide it out from behind you as you keep your legs up. Practice until you can no longer pull the towel out from behind you.

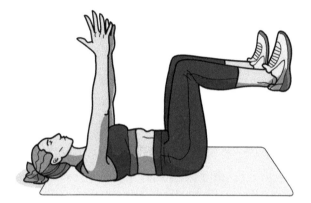

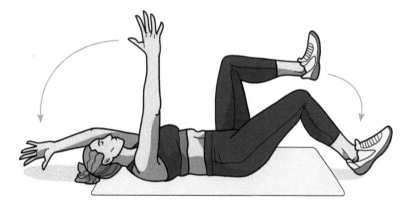

RUSSIAN TWIST

ADDITIONAL MUSCLES WORKED: *Arms, Quads*

This move targets your obliques and lower abs really well. It's also a good way to train your body to rotate from the T-spine, as opposed to your lower back, which protects your lower back.

1. Sit on the floor with your feet together and knees bent. Hold a dumbbell at your chest with both hands.

2. Lean back slightly and lift your feet off the ground.

3. Twist using your T-spine and obliques instead of just your arms to rotate the weight to the right side of your torso. Rotate back through your center and to the left. Rotate your head so that your eyes can follow the weight.

4. Continue rotating side to side. Keep your legs from moving side to side as you do this.

Lift Safely: Make sure to relax your neck and shoulders and keep your back straight the entire time. Twist from the middle of your back, not your lower back.

Make It Easier: Keep your feet on the ground. You can also make it easier by not using a weight and just work at getting the side-to-side motion down.

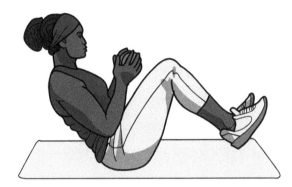

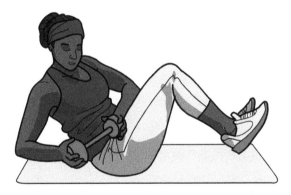

COBRA

Just like other muscle groups, your abs can cramp up. You want to stretch them out between sets to avoid this. Cobra is a great way to accomplish this as it stretches the front of your body.

1. Lie on your stomach with your arms bent and your hands next to your chest. Keep your feet together with the tops of your feet pressed into the ground.

2. Press your hands into the floor and raise your chest off the ground as you extend your elbows. Your hips should remain in contact with the ground as you do this.

3. Stop extending your back when you feel a good stretch in your abs and no discomfort in your lower back. Release and lower back to the floor.

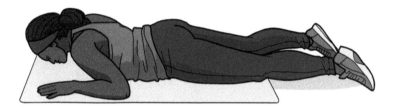

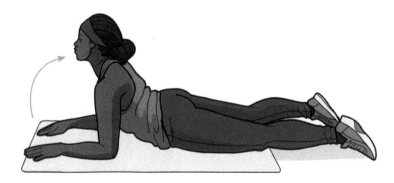

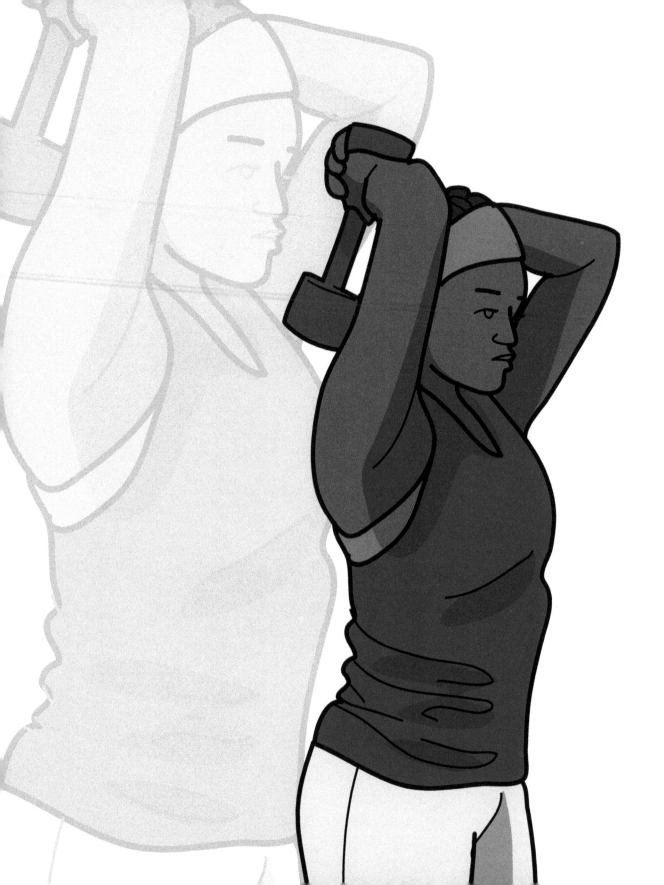

9. BICEPS AND TRICEPS

While your arms are made up of many muscles, the biceps and triceps are the muscles that most people think of when talking about weight training. Some women feel like they have weak arms but fear lifting weights because they don't want to get "bulky." It takes a very specific style of training for your arms and a very specific way of eating (which involves a lot of calories) for women to get bulky. This applies to a woman's body in general but is also true of the arms specifically. Weightlifting will help you tone your arms and gain more strength. Do you want to be able to carry items with ease and comfort or convincingly flex your arms as you tell someone they have 3 seconds to back away from you? If your answer is yes to either of these scenarios, this is the chapter for you.

The biceps are the muscles of your arms that face the front when your arms are at rest at your sides. The triceps are the muscle group in the back of your arms when your arms are at rest. You have two bicep heads and three tricep heads. This is why one group is named "bi-" and the other "tri-." The two heads of the biceps (biceps brachii) are the long head and the short head. The long head and short head originate from two different points of the scapula to assist in slightly different movements. The three heads of the triceps (triceps brachii) are the long head, lateral head, and medial head. The lateral and medial heads originate from different points on the humerus (arm bone), and the long head originates from the scapula. This means that each tricep head moves the arm slightly different from another. The biceps and triceps work opposite of each other. Biceps flex your elbow, and the triceps extend your elbow. This means that your biceps and triceps are active whenever you do any type of push or pull movement, such as push-ups, chest presses, pull-ups, and rows. It's more effective to work your arms as a part of working a larger muscle group, as you'll burn more calories using large muscle groups. However, if you are specifically looking to build extra definition in your arms, then it is recommended that you do a few isolated arm exercises.

Before You Lift:

Remember to keep your core engaged while executing the movements in this chapter. You can also perform each of these movements in front of a mirror, or record yourself, to double-check your form.

UP-DOWN PLANK

This movement is a great way to increase your heart rate and get blood flowing to your arms. The up-and-down movement will help prepare your arms for your weightlifting sets.

1. Begin in a low plank position on the floor with your elbows directly under your shoulders and your toes on the ground, hip-width apart.

2. Walk yourself up onto your right hand, as you leave your left forearm on the ground. You should be in a half push-up position.

3. Walk up onto your left hand so that you are now in the top of a push-up position with both hands on the ground under your shoulders.

4. Lower one arm back to the ground so that you are on one forearm once again.

5. Lower the other arm down so that both forearms are on the ground and you're back in a low plank position.

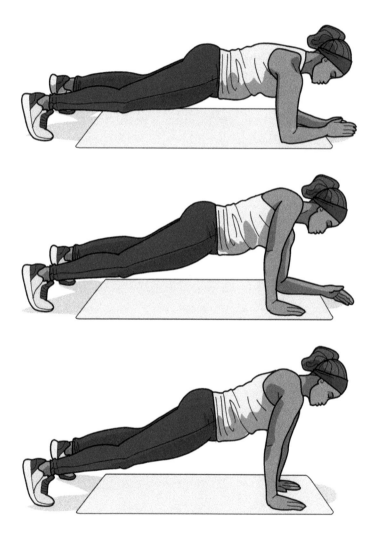

TRADITIONAL BICEP CURL

ADDITIONAL MUSCLES WORKED: *Forearms*

This type of curl is great for developing extra definition and strength specifically in the biceps of each arm. It's also great for increasing the strength in your biceps so that you can lift heavier weights when performing back exercises.

1. Stand with your feet hip-width apart, holding a barbell in front of you at your thighs, palms up. You can also use dumbbells for this movement. Hold the dumbbells at your sides.

2. Slowly bend your elbows and raise the weight up toward your chest. Stop just in front of your chest.

3. Extend at your elbows to lower the weight back down to tap your thighs.

Lift Safely: Relax your shoulders and neck as you perform this exercise. Keep your elbows at your sides throughout the movement. They shouldn't shift forward or back. In addition, it is important that you stand with your knees slightly bent and not locked, in order to avoid circulation issues.

Make It Harder: Take 1 second to bring the weight up and then 3 seconds to bring the weight back down. The reason for taking more time to lower the weight is that you build more muscle on the downward movement. Alternatively, use dumbbells to isolate each arm. If you are using dumbbells, externally rotating the dumbbells as you curl will better target both the short (inner) and long (outer) heads of the bicep muscles and activate more muscle fibers, which builds more muscle.

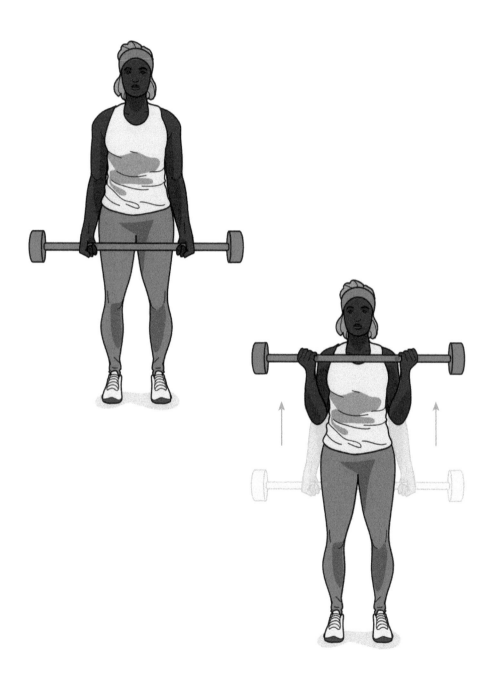

HAMMER CURL

ADDITIONAL MUSCLES WORKED: *Forearms*

Hammer Curls work a different part of your biceps than Traditional Bicep Curls. They target the long heads of the biceps, the brachioradialis (a forearm muscle in charge of external rotation), and the brachialis, which is another muscle that sits in the arm but is different from the biceps. Hammer Curls will help your biceps build more strength and size while also strengthening your wrists.

1. Stand with your feet hip-width apart with a dumbbell in each hand at your side and with your palms facing inward.

2. Bend your elbows and raise both weights up until they reach your chest. Keep your palms facing inward toward each other. (The movement is the same motion you would use to raise a glass for a drink.)

3. Lower the weights back down to your sides.

Lift Safely: It is important that you stand with your knees slightly bent and not locked in order to avoid circulation issues.

Make It Easier: Lift one arm at a time. Doing this will feel easier than when you try to lift both at the same time.

Make It Harder: Take 1 second to lift the weights and 3 seconds to bring them back down.

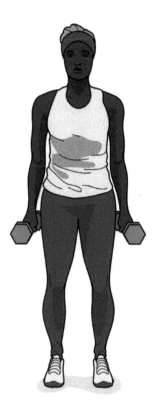

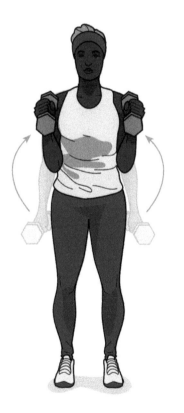

TRICEP KICKBACK

ADDITIONAL MUSCLES WORKED: *Forearms*

This is an excellent exercise that targets the backs of the arms. Isolating the work in each arm with dumbbells means neither side is compensating for the other, and you may notice that your triceps muscles are stronger in one arm.

1. Stand with your feet hip-width apart and your knees slightly bent. Hold the dumbbells at your sides with palms facing inward toward your thighs.

2. Hinge from your hips and drop your chest down slightly. Hold this position, looking a few feet in front of you at the floor to keep your spine long.

3. Bend your elbows and, at the same time, bring your elbows up behind you so that the weights are up next to your upper ribs.

4. Extend your elbows straight back without lifting your chest or moving your shoulders to bring the dumbbells toward the ceiling.

5. Flex your elbows to bring the weights back to their starting position.

Make It Easier: Lift one weight at a time instead of trying to do both at the same time.

Make It Harder: Hold your position for 1 second once you've extended your elbows fully before releasing. You can also slow the movement down to make it more challenging.

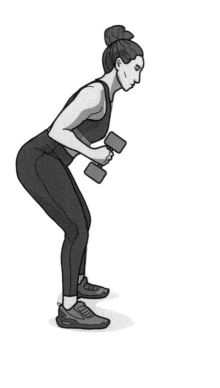

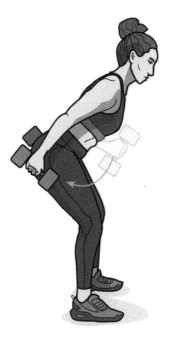

TRICEP OVERHEAD EXTENSION

ADDITIONAL MUSCLES WORKED: *Forearms, Shoulders*

By extending your arms overhead for this exercise, you target your triceps muscles in a different way and work the shoulders a bit more by holding them in place. This movement will also help improve your shoulder mobility. However, if you have a shoulder injury or lack of mobility, choose one of the other triceps exercises mentioned.

1. Stand with your feet shoulder-width apart.

2. Extend your arms overhead, holding one weight in both hands by making a diamond shape between the palms of your hands.

3. Bend your elbows so that the weight comes directly behind your head.

4. Straighten your elbows to bring the weight back overhead.

Lift Safely: Do not arch your back while performing this exercise, and keep your rib cage down. (Think about not puffing out your chest.)

Make It Harder: Add a 2-second hold at the top of the movement before lowering the weight back down behind your head.

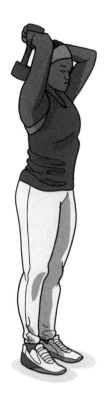

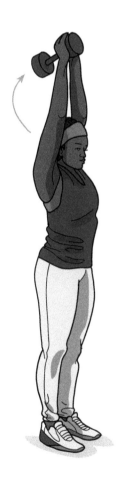

OVERHEAD PULL

ADDITIONAL MUSCLES WORKED: *Core, Shoulders*

This is an excellent exercise for improving your shoulder mobility and core stability as you work your triceps. It's three great benefits in one movement!

1. Lie on the ground on your back with your knees bent and feet flat on the floor.

2. Hold one weight above your chest by extending your elbows and making a diamond shape between the palms of your hands.

3. Bend your elbows slightly, then extend the weight back overhead as far as you can go without allowing your lower back to arch or your rib cage to lift up.

4. Pull the weight forward to bring it back over your chest and return the shoulders to the starting position.

Lift Safely: Do not let your lower back arch while performing this exercise, and be sure not to overextend your shoulders. Only work within a comfortable range of motion until your shoulder mobility improves.

Make It Harder: Bring your knees over your hips and lift your feet off the ground. This will require more core stability.

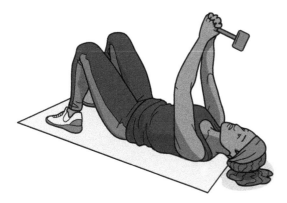

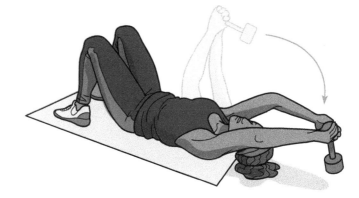

STANDING BICEP STRETCH

This is one way to stretch your biceps so that you don't catch a cramp following your isolated weightlifting. You may notice your elbows staying in a bent position after a bicep workout because your biceps have shortened. It's important to stretch your biceps to restore them to their original length. Tight, shortened biceps can cause your shoulders to round forward, which in turn will affect your shoulder mobility.

1. Stand with your feet hip-width apart.

2. Place your hands behind your back, interlace your fingers, and rotate your elbows inward to move your palms into a ground-facing position.

3. Extend your shoulders and raise your arms up behind you until you feel a stretch in your biceps.

4. Return your hands to the starting position.

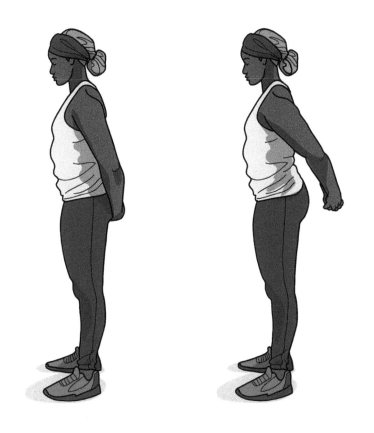

OVERHEAD TRICEP STRETCH

Perform this stretch directly following a triceps workout to avoid cramps in the back of your arms. You'll also want to do this stretch to avoid tennis elbow—this is pain felt in the elbow joint due to overusing the forearms or performing repetitive elbow flexion movements.

1. Stand with your feet hip-width apart.

2. Reach one arm overhead and bend that elbow so that your hand is close to your shoulder.

3. Reach the opposite arm up and press down and back on the elbow of the bent arm until you feel a nice stretch in the triceps.

4. Release and repeat on the opposite side.

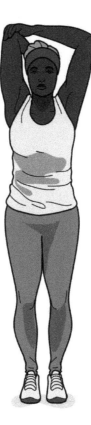

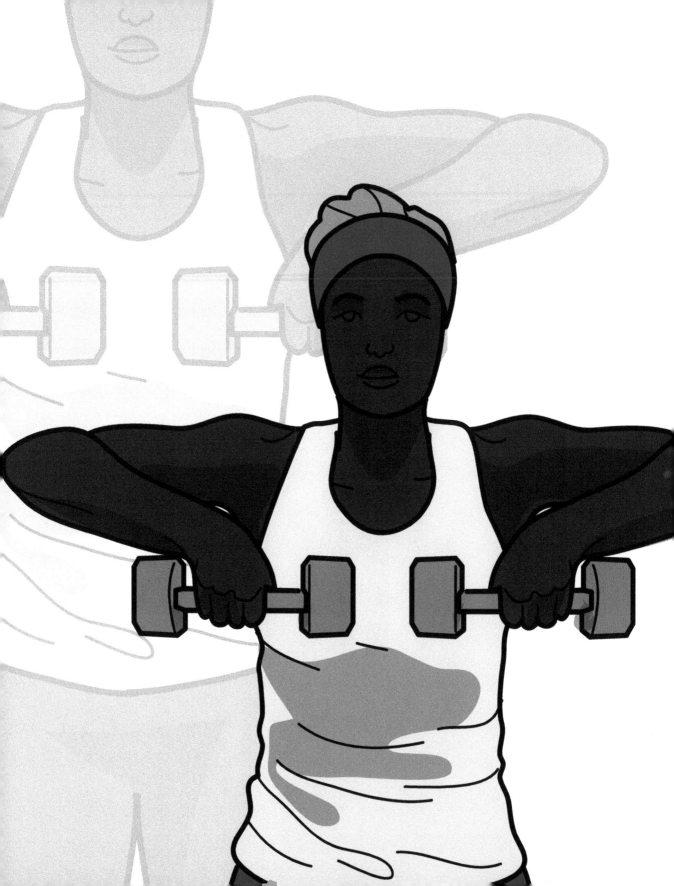

10. SHOULDERS

The shoulders are a powerful but sensitive muscle group. The muscles in the shoulder girdle include the rotator cuff muscles, trapezius, rhomboids, serratus anterior, levator scapulae, and pectoralis minor. Many people think that the deltoids are the only muscles of the shoulder, but that is not true. There are many other muscles that act on the shoulder joint, including the latissimus dorsi, commonly referred to as the "lats." Each of these muscles acts to move your shoulder in one of the following ways: flexion, extension, internal rotation, external rotation, adduction, and abduction. As you can see, the shoulder is a complex area that requires a lot of synergy within the body.

Due to the shallowness of the ball-and-socket joint of your shoulder, the shoulder joints don't have as much bony support as your hip joint (the other ball-and-socket joint in your body). Therefore, the shoulder needs more muscular support to maintain its stability. Without that muscular support, the shoulder is prone to injuries such as dislocation. Furthermore, most people have internally rotated shoulders as a result of sitting for prolonged periods of time. This restricts the range of motion that the shoulder should naturally have and therefore puts the shoulder joint at more risk for injury. Thus, it is very important to work on your shoulder mobility and also the stability of the muscles supporting the shoulder joint. Mobility precedes stability. That means you'll want to work on making sure you have full shoulder range of motion before beginning your weightlifting routine–one way to do this is by warming up the shoulders with the warm-up movements in this chapter.

Before You Lift:

Remember to keep your core engaged while executing the movements in this chapter. You can also perform each of these movements in front of a mirror, or record yourself, to double-check your form.

CROSS-BODY ARM SWING

This movement will help increase blood flow to your shoulder joint. Before performing any shoulder exercises, you want to make sure your joints are sufficiently lubricated to avoid injury.

1. Stand with your feet hip-width apart and your arms straight out to your sides in a T-formation.

2. Swing your arms forward so that one arm crosses in front of the other in the center of your body.

3. Return your arms to the outstretched, open position. Repeat, swinging your arms forward, then back out to your sides at chest height.

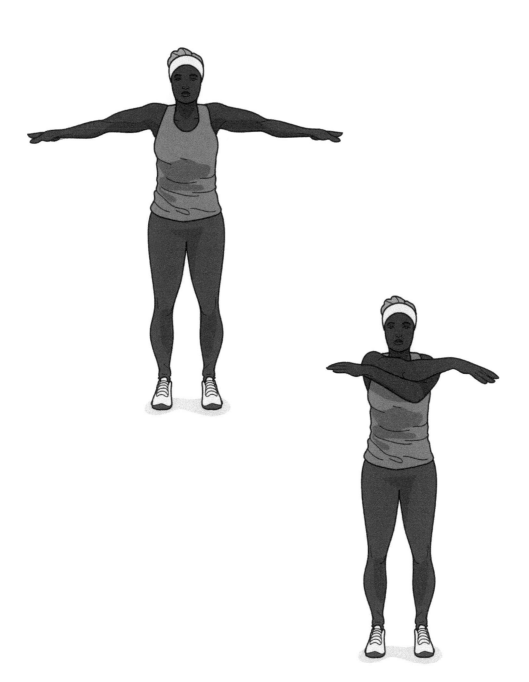

WALL ANGEL

This stretch is very helpful for increasing your shoulder mobility. It also helps combat the internal rotation of the shoulder (also known as rounding) that most people have as a result of sitting most of the day.

1. Stand against a wall with your butt in contact with the wall and your rib cage down.

2. Bring your arms up onto the wall, with your elbows at shoulder height and bent at a 90-degree angle, creating a goal post with your arms.

3. Slowly reach your arms up while trying to maintain contact with the wall until your elbows are straight and your hands are above your head.

4. Lower your hands back down so that you return to the starting position with your elbows at a 90-degree angle.

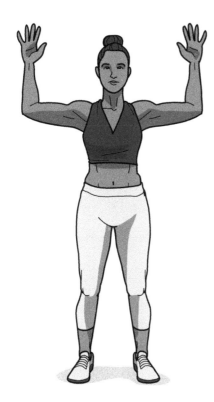

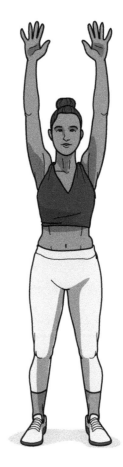

SHOULDER PRESS

ADDITIONAL MUSCLES WORKED: *Biceps*

This movement is one of the fundamental movement patterns that humans develop from birth. It's one of the most common vertical press movements but should not be performed if you have a shoulder injury or have limited range of motion in your shoulders.

1. Stand with your feet shoulder-width apart holding dumbbells in your hands, or a barbell in both hands, and palms out.

2. Bring your elbows to shoulder height and align your wrists above your elbows, creating a 90-degree angle with your elbows.

3. Press the weights above your head and fully extend the elbows.

4. Return your arms to the starting position.

Lift Safely: Do not arch your lower back as you press the weights into the air. Keep your rib cage down and your neck neutral as you press the weights overhead.

Make It Easier: Press one dumbbell at a time into the air to require less core engagement.

Home Workout Hack: Perform this exercise using a resistance band. Simply stand on the band and press the handles over your head. Standing on the band with two feet will create more resistance than if you stand on the band with one foot.

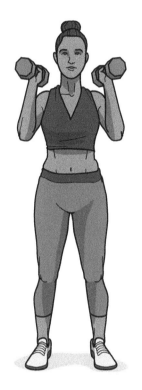

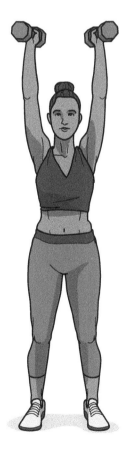

IRON CROSS

ADDITIONAL MUSCLES WORKED: *Forearms*

This exercise is very effective for working all three heads of your deltoid muscle, which is found in the top of your shoulder.

1. Stand with your feet shoulder-width apart holding the dumbbells in front of you and your palms down.

2. Raise your arms straight up in front of you to bring the dumbbells to shoulder height.

3. Keeping the dumbbells at shoulder height, extend your arms laterally (out to your sides) to form a T.

4. Lower both arms straight back down to the sides of your body.

5. Raise your arms straight up laterally, stopping when your hands are at the same height as your shoulders, to form that T.

6. Keeping the dumbbells at shoulder height, bring your arms together in the center of your body while keeping your arms straight.

7. Lower both arms back down along the front of your torso to bring the dumbbells back to the starting position.

Life Safely: Do not arch your lower back as you perform this movement. Do not raise your hands past the height of your shoulders at any point during this exercise.

Home Workout Hack: You can use resistance bands to perform this movement.

Make It Easier: Perform lateral raises and/or front raises instead of the full Iron Cross. Front raises are the first part of the movement. (Raise the weights to shoulder height and then lower them back down to your waist.) Lateral raises are the second half of the movement. (Raise your arms laterally with a slight bend in your elbows and then lower the weights back down by your sides.)

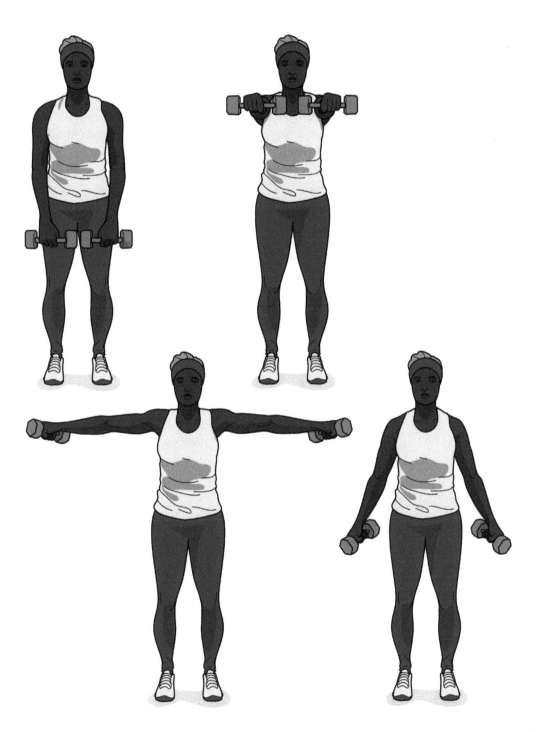

UPRIGHT ROW

ADDITIONAL MUSCLES WORKED: *Biceps*

This exercise targets small muscle groups of the shoulder that are different from the ones worked in the previous two exercises. It is a frontal plane movement that focuses more on the front and middle of your shoulders. This movement is popular among bodybuilders to help create more definition in the shoulders. It is not recommended if you don't have good posture or healthy shoulders. Consider a more functional exercise, like the ones mention previously, if you have any contraindications.

1. Stand with your feet shoulder-width apart holding dumbbells, or a barbell, in front of your body at your thighs, hands shoulder-width apart, and with your palms turned toward your body.

2. Raise the weights up to the height of your chest by bending your elbows. Imagine yourself trying to create the shape of a clothes hanger with your elbows.

3. Return your arms to the starting position, keeping the weights close to your body throughout the movement.

Lift Safely: Do not arch your lower back as you perform this exercise. Stop if you feel any pinching or discomfort in the front of your shoulder. Think about squeezing your shoulder blades together on your back as you raise the weights up to chest height—similar to a wide row. This will help reduce some of the strain caused by the internal rotation of the shoulders.

Make It Easier: Lift one dumbbell at a time instead of simultaneously.

Home Workout Hack: You can do this exercise with a resistance band.

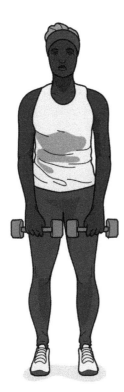

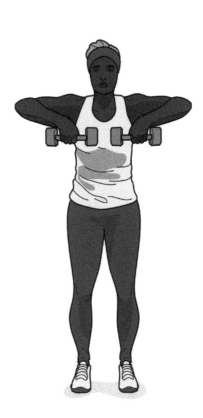

CROSS-BODY STRETCH

Just as it is important to warm up the shoulder joint, it is important to stretch out the joint post-workout to return the muscles to their original lengths. This will help you maintain proper joint range of motion.

1. Stand with your arms at your sides.

2. Raise one arm up and cross it to the other side of your body while keeping the arm straight.

3. Take the opposite hand and grasp the arm crossing your body just beyond the elbow.

4. Pull the arm toward your torso so that you feel a stretch in your shoulder and triceps.

5. Release and repeat on the opposite side.

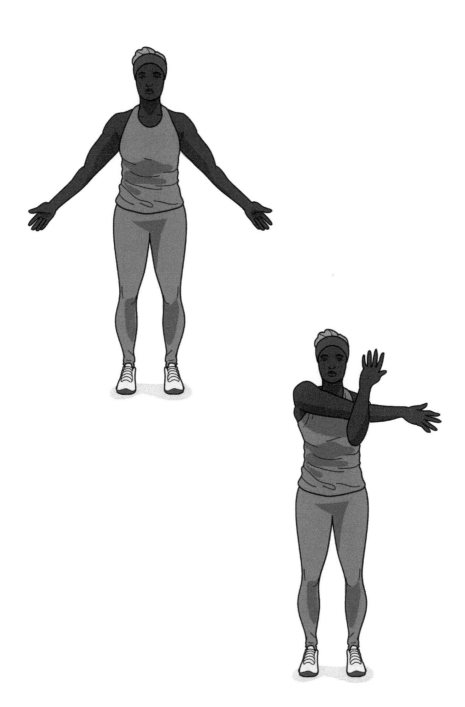

WORKOUT PROGRAMS

This is where I bring together all the elements for you to build and experience successful workouts. It is important to have a program to follow when working out so that you can keep track of your weightlifting progress. It also keeps you focused on the exercise movements during your workout so that you aren't stressing about what to do next. Over the next few pages, you will find the tools for building your own workouts (called programming); information on reps, sets, and exercise tempo; and example weekly programming and various sample workouts for your total body, upper body, and lower body that you can use to get started or to inform building your own workout program.

Programming

Programming is a very complex process. I strongly suggest that you seek the guidance of a certified personal trainer to assist you in creating a fitness program that works best for you. This is important because there are many different ways to program and it can be difficult for a beginner to sort out which types of programs would work best for you and your goals. Once you've been evaluated by a fitness professional, you'll have a better starting point for learning how to create and apply your own programs.

For the purpose of this book, I have created sample programs under the assumption that you should circuit train and incorporate supersets for maximum fat burning and strength training. For upper-body exercises, I recommend separating exercises into vertical pushes, vertical pulls, horizontal pushes, and horizontal pulls. This will help ensure that you work every muscle group. With some muscle groups it's a little difficult to fit into this strict mold; however, you'll start to learn which muscles are commonly working with each movement pattern and the classifications will make more sense. For example, a Shoulder Press would be a vertical push. However, an Upright Row is still a shoulder exercise but is a vertical pull. So that's where the rule gets a little tricky.

For lower-body exercises, it is recommended that you split your movements into knee-dominant and hip-dominant exercises. Knee-dominant exercises are generally movements where your knee bends and extends. Hip-dominant exercises are movements that usually require hip flexion and extension, like movements where you hinge at the hips. I've also included total-body workouts for those who can only train a few days a week.

Reps, Sets, and Tempo

For building strength, it is recommended you perform 3 to 5 sets of 5 to 8 reps for each exercise. The tempo should be about 3 seconds up and 3 seconds down for each exercise. Make sure to take 90 seconds to 2 minutes of rest after each set.

Progression

As you progress through your workouts, you'll want to change things up a bit each week. For example, if in week 1 you started with 3 sets of 5 reps, in week 2 you can do 3 sets of 8. Alternatively, you could stick with 3 sets of 5, but increase the weight. You want to change the sets, reps, tempo, or amount of rest each week to make sure that you are not plateauing in your strength training program. It is also important that you only change one thing at a time. If you try to change too many factors at once, you will confuse your body, and this will cause issues in its ability to adapt and get stronger.

Equipment

For each of the exercises and subsequent workout programs in this book, you will want to have a set of medium and a set of heavy dumbbells, as well as a barbell that you can add or remove weight from, if you're planning to build strength. Medium weights should feel like you could maybe do 3 to 5 more reps if needed. Heavy weights should feel like you could only maybe do 1 or 2 more reps. While many of these movements can be done with body weight to regress (or make them easier), free weights allow you to progressively increase your load to work your muscles harder.

Rest and Recovery Days

It is recommended to take a day or two off in between each workout for proper rest and muscle recovery. Once you get used to weightlifting and have a better idea of programming, you can begin to work out on consecutive days. You'll still want at least 1 recovery day per week, and you'll want to take 2 days of rest per muscle group if possible.

Warm-Ups and Cooldowns

As mentioned in the beginning of this book, warm-ups and cooldowns should not be skipped. Warming up and cooling down are essential for helping your body recover and for preventing injuries. I've included warm-up and cooldown moves in the programs provided later in the book.

Scheduling

On the next few pages, I've included a few examples of what your week of workouts could look like based on your training availability. You'll notice I've included rest days and cardio options on non–weight training days. You can use these examples as a template to structure your weeks in whatever way works best for your schedule. I recommend sitting down one evening a week—perhaps Sunday night before a new week begins—and scheduling out your week of workouts. This will help you remain accountable to yourself and your training, as well as ensure that you block out specific time for training so that nothing unexpected pops up and leaves you with no time to work out.

For those who can commit to 3 days of training per week:

EXAMPLE 1:

Monday: Upper-Body Workout 2 (page 159)
Tuesday: Cardio (walk, run, bike, etc.)
Wednesday: Lower-Body Workout 1 (page 162)
Thursday: Rest Day
Friday: Total-Body Workout 1 (page 154)
Saturday: Cardio
Sunday: Rest Day

EXAMPLE 2:

Monday: Lower-Body Workout 2 (page 163)
Tuesday: Rest Day
Wednesday: Upper-Body Workout 3 (page 161)
Thursday: Cardio
Friday: Total-Body Workout 2 (page 155)
Saturday: Rest Day
Sunday: Cardio

EXAMPLE 3:

Monday: Total-Body Workout 3 (page 157)
Tuesday: Cardio
Wednesday: Upper-Body Workout 1 (page 158)
Thursday: Cardio
Friday: Lower-Body Workout 3 (page 164)
Saturday: Rest Day
Sunday: Rest Day

For those who can commit to 4 days of training per week:

EXAMPLE:

Monday: Upper-Body Workout 1 (page 158)
Tuesday: Lower-Body Workout 1 (page 162)
Wednesday: Cardio
Thursday: Upper-Body Workout 2 (page 159)
Friday: Lower-Body Workout 2 (page 163)
Saturday: Rest Day
Sunday: Rest Day

For those who can commit to 5 days of training per week:

EXAMPLE:

Monday: Total-Body Workout 3 (page 157)
Tuesday: Shoulders and Core*
Wednesday: Lower-Body Workout 3 (page 164)
Thursday: Back and Arms*
Friday: Cardio
Saturday: Lower-Body Workout 2 (page 163)
Sunday: Rest Day

*Use the exercises from earlier chapters and follow the programming information in this book to practice building your own workouts, including the number of sets and reps, tempo, and rest time between sets. Don't forget to include warm-up movements before you lift and stretches to finish out your workout program.

Total-Body Workouts

TOTAL-BODY WORKOUT 1

WARM-UP

Sets: 1
Reps: Perform each move for 30 to 60 seconds
Rest: No rest between moves
Tempo: Fast
Equipment: None

- Butt Kicker (page 48)
- World's Greatest Stretch (page 28)
- Wall Angel (page 140)
- Straight-Leg Kick (page 26)

WORKOUT

Sets: 3 to 5
Reps: 5 to 8
Rest: 1 to 2 minutes between sets
Instructions: Perform 3 to 5 sets of each exercise and then move on to the next exercise for optimal strength gains. If you want to superset muscle groups, then you can perform 1 set of an exercise and then go straight to the next exercise. Repeat that pattern for 3 to 5 sets total. Performing supersets will increase the fat-burning effects of strength training.
Tempo: Moderate (about 3 seconds each direction)
Equipment: Medium to heavy dumbbells, barbell

- Horizontal Push: Wide-Grip Barbell Chest Press (page 76)
- Horizontal Pull: Bent-Over Row (page 84)
- Vertical Push: Shoulder Press (page 142)
- Vertical Pull: Overhead Pull (page 130)
- Hip Dominant: Deadlift (page 30)
- Knee Dominant: Goblet Squat (page 50)
- Core: Plank (page 104)

COOLDOWN

Sets: 1
Reps: Perform each stretch for 30 to 60 seconds
Rest: No rest between moves
Tempo: Slow
Equipment: None

- Standing Quad Stretch (page 66)
- Wall Stretch (page 78)
- Child's Pose (page 100)

TOTAL-BODY WORKOUT 2

WARM-UP

Sets: 1
Reps: Perform each move for 30 to 60 seconds
Rest: No rest between moves
Tempo: Fast
Equipment: None

- World's Greatest Stretch (page 28)
- Scaption Plank (page 70)
- T-Spine Rotation (page 82)
- Plank (page 104)

WORKOUT

Sets: 3 to 5
Reps: 5 to 8
Rest: 1 to 2 minutes between sets
Instructions: Perform 3 to 5 sets of each exercise and then move on to the next exercise for optimal strength gains. If you want to superset muscle groups, then you can perform 1 set of an exercise and then go straight to the next exercise. Repeat that pattern for 3 to 5 sets total. Performing supersets will increase the fat-burning effects of strength training.
Tempo: Moderate (about 3 seconds each direction)
Equipment: Medium to heavy dumbbells, barbell

- Horizontal Push: Dumbbell Chest Fly (page 74)
- Horizontal Pull: Reverse Fly (page 86)
- Vertical Press: Upright Row (page 146)
- Vertical Pull: Dumbbell Bird-Dog (page 96)
- Hip Dominant: Single-Leg Romanian Deadlift (page 32)
- Knee Dominant: Forward Lunge (page 52)
- Core: Side Bridge (page 106)

COOLDOWN

Sets: 1
Reps: Perform each stretch for 30 to 60 seconds
Rest: No rest between moves
Tempo: Slow
Equipment: None

- Pretzel Stretch (page 42)
- Seated Toe Touch (page 44)
- Cat-Cow (page 90)

TOTAL-BODY WORKOUT 3

WARM-UP

Sets: 1
Reps: Perform each move for 30 to 60 seconds
Rest: No rest between moves
Tempo: Fast
Equipment: None

- Straight-Leg Kick (page 26)
- Butt Kicker (page 48)
- T-Spine Rotation (page 82)
- Up-Down Plank (page 120)

WORKOUT

Sets: 3 to 5
Reps: 5 to 8
Rest: 1 to 2 minutes between sets
Instructions: Perform 3 to 5 sets of each exercise and then move on to the next exercise for optimal strength gains. If you want to superset muscle groups, then you can perform 1 set of an exercise and then go straight to the next exercise. Repeat that pattern for 3 to 5 sets total. Performing supersets will increase the fat-burning effects of strength training.
Tempo: Moderate (about 3 seconds each direction)
Equipment: Medium to heavy dumbbells, barbell

- Horizontal Push: Wide-Grip Barbell Chest Press (page 76)
- Horizontal Pull: Bent-Over Row (page 84)
- Vertical Push: Iron Cross (page 144)
- Lower Back/Vertical Pull: Good Morning (page 98)
- Hip Dominant: Glute Bridge (page 34)
- Knee Dominant: Lateral Lunge (page 54)
- Core: Hollow-Body Hold (page 108)

COOLDOWN

Sets: 1
Reps: Perform each stretch for 30 to 60 seconds
Rest: No rest between moves
Tempo: Slow
Equipment: None

- Cross-Body Stretch (page 148)
- Cat-Cow (page 90)
- Cobra (page 116)
- Standing Quad Stretch (page 66)

Upper-Body Workouts

UPPER-BODY WORKOUT 1 (BACK AND BICEPS)

WARM-UP

Sets: 1
Reps: Perform each move for 30 to 60 seconds
Rest: No rest between moves
Tempo: Fast
Equipment: None

- Cross-Body Arm Swing (page 138)
- Up-Down Plank (page 120)
- Scaption Plank (page 70)
- T-Spine Rotation (page 82)

WORKOUT

Sets: 3 to 5
Reps: 5 to 8
Rest: 1 to 2 minutes between sets
Instructions: Perform 3 to 5 sets of each exercise and then move on to the next exercise for optimal strength gains. If you want to superset muscle groups, then you can perform 1 set of an exercise and then go straight to the next exercise. Repeat that pattern for 3 to 5 sets total. Performing supersets will increase the fat-burning effects of strength training.

Tempo: Moderate (about 3 seconds each direction)
Equipment: Medium to heavy dumbbells, barbell

- Bent-Over Row (page 84)
- Reverse Fly (page 86)
- Farmer's Carry (page 88)
- Good Morning (page 98)
- Traditional Bicep Curl (page 122)
- Hammer Curl (page 124)

COOLDOWN

Sets: 1
Reps: Perform each stretch for 30 to 60 seconds
Rest: No rest between moves
Tempo: Slow
Equipment: None

- Standing Bicep Stretch (page 132)
- Cat-Cow (page 90)
- Child's Pose (page 100)

UPPER-BODY WORKOUT 2 (TOTAL UPPER BODY)

WARM-UP

Sets: 1
Reps: Perform each move for 30 to 60 seconds
Rest: No rest between moves
Tempo: Fast
Equipment: None

- Cross-Body Arm Swing (page 138)
- Up-Down Plank (page 120)
- Scaption Plank (page 70)
- T-Spine Rotation (page 82)

WORKOUT

Sets: 3 to 5
Reps: 5 to 8
Rest: 1 to 2 minutes between sets
Instructions: Perform 3 to 5 sets of each exercise and then move on to the next exercise for optimal strength gains. If you want to superset muscle groups, then you can perform 1 set of an exercise and then go straight to the next exercise. Repeat that pattern for 3 to 5 sets total. Performing supersets will increase the fat-burning effects of strength training.
Tempo: Moderate (about 3 seconds each direction)
Equipment: Medium to heavy dumbbells, barbell

- Chest: Dumbbell Chest Fly (page 74)
- Back: Farmer's Carry (page 88)
- Shoulders: Iron Cross (page 144)
- Biceps: Hammer Curl (page 124)
- Triceps: Tricep Overhead Extension (page 128)

COOLDOWN

Sets: 1
Reps: Perform each stretch for 30 to 60 seconds
Rest: No rest between moves
Tempo: Slow
Equipment: None

- Cat-Cow (page 90)
- Child's Pose (page 100)
- T-Spine Rotation (page 82)
- Wall Stretch (page 78)

UPPER-BODY WORKOUT 3 (CHEST AND TRICEPS)

WARM-UP

Sets: 1
Reps: Perform each move for 30 seconds
Rest: No rest between moves
Tempo: Fast
Equipment: None

- Cross-Body Arm Swing (page 138)
- Up-Down Plank (page 120)
- T-Spine Rotation (page 82)

WORKOUT

Sets: 3 to 5
Reps: 5 to 8
Rest: 1 to 2 minutes between sets
Instructions: Perform 3 to 5 sets of each exercise and then move on to the next exercise for optimal strength gains. If you want to superset muscle groups, then you can perform 1 set of an exercise and then go straight to the next exercise. Repeat that pattern for 3 to 5 sets total. Performing supersets will increase the fat-burning effects of strength training.
Tempo: Moderate (about 3 seconds each direction)
Equipment: Medium to heavy dumbbells, barbell

- Wide-Grip Barbell Chest Press (page 76)
- Dumbbell Chest Fly (page 74)
- Dumbbell Floor Press (page 72)
- Tricep Kickback (page 126)
- Tricep Overhead Extension (page 128)

Sets: 1
Reps: Perform each stretch for 30 to 60 seconds
Rest: No rest between moves
Tempo: Slow
Equipment: None

- Overhead Tricep Stretch (page 134)
- Wall Stretch (page 78)
- Child's Pose (page 100)

Lower-Body Workouts

LOWER-BODY WORKOUT 1 (HIP DOMINANT)

WARM-UP

Sets: 1
Reps: Perform each move for 30 to 60 seconds
Rest: No rest between moves
Tempo: Fast
Equipment: None

- Straight-Leg Kick (page 26)
- World's Greatest Stretch (page 28)
- Butt Kicker (page 48)
- Plank (page 104)

WORKOUT

Sets: 3 to 5
Reps: 5 to 8
Rest: 1 to 2 minutes between sets
Instructions: Perform 3 to 5 sets of each exercise and then move on to the next exercise for optimal strength gains. If you want to superset muscle groups, then you can perform 1 set of an exercise and then go straight to the next exercise. Repeat that pattern for 3 to 5 sets total. Performing supersets will increase the fat-burning effects of strength training.

Tempo: Moderate (about 3 seconds each direction)
Equipment: Medium to heavy dumbbells, barbell

- Step-Up (page 38)
- Deadlift (page 30)
- Single-Leg Glute Bridge (page 36)
- Single-Leg Romanian Deadlift (page 32)

COOLDOWN

Sets: 1
Reps: Perform each stretch for 30 to 60 seconds
Rest: No rest between moves
Tempo: Slow
Equipment: None

- Pretzel Stretch (page 42)
- Seated Toe Touch (page 44)
- Standing Calf Stretch (page 64)

LOWER-BODY WORKOUT 2 (KNEE DOMINANT)

WARM-UP

Sets: 1
Reps: Perform each move for 30 to 60 seconds
Rest: No rest between moves
Tempo: Fast
Equipment: None

- Straight-Leg Kick (page 26)
- World's Greatest Stretch (page 28)
- Butt Kicker (page 48)
- Plank (page 104)

WORKOUT

Sets: 3 to 5
Reps: 5 to 8
Rest: 1 to 2 minutes between sets
Instructions: Perform 3 to 5 sets of each exercise and then move on to the next exercise for optimal strength gains. If you want to superset muscle groups, then you can perform 1 set of an exercise and then go straight to the next exercise. Repeat that pattern for 3 to 5 sets total. Performing supersets will increase the fat-burning effects of strength training.
Tempo: Moderate (about 3 seconds each direction)
Equipment: Medium to heavy dumbbells, barbell

- Goblet Squat (page 50)
- Forward Lunge (page 52)
- Lateral Lunge (page 54)
- Suitcase Squat (page 58)
- Single-Leg Goblet Squat (page 60)

COOLDOWN

Sets: 1
Reps: Perform each stretch for 30 to 60 seconds
Rest: No rest between moves
Tempo: Slow
Equipment: None

- Pretzel Stretch (page 42)
- Seated Toe Touch (page 44)
- Standing Quad Stretch (page 66)

LOWER-BODY WORKOUT 3 (TOTAL LOWER BODY)

WARM-UP

Sets: 1
Reps: Perform each move for 30 to 60 seconds
Rest: No rest between moves
Tempo: Fast
Equipment: None

- Straight-Leg Kick (page 26)
- World's Greatest Stretch (page 28)
- Butt Kicker (page 48)
- Plank (page 104)

WORKOUT

Sets: 3 to 5

Reps: 5 to 8

Rest: 1 to 2 minutes between sets

Instructions: Perform 3 to 5 sets of each exercise and then move on to the next exercise for optimal strength gains. If you want to superset muscle groups, then you can perform 1 set of an exercise and then go straight to the next exercise. Repeat that pattern for 3 to 5 sets total. Performing supersets will increase the fat-burning effects of strength training.

Tempo: Moderate (about 3 seconds each direction)

Equipment: Medium to heavy dumbbells, barbell

- Lateral Step-Up (page 40)
- Deadlift (page 30)
- Curtsy Lunge (page 62)
- Bulgarian Split Squat (page 56)

COOLDOWN

Sets: 1

Reps: Perform each stretch for 30 to 60 seconds

Rest: No rest between moves

Tempo: Slow

Equipment: None

- Pretzel Stretch (page 42)
- Seated Toe Touch (page 44)
- Standing Calf Stretch (page 64)
- Standing Quad Stretch (page 66)

GLOSSARY

abduction: The action of moving a limb away from the midline of the body.

adduction: The action of moving a limb back toward the midline of the body.

biceps: The muscles in the front part of the upper arm.

calves: The muscles in the back of the lower leg.

core: The muscles of the midsection that are responsible for stabilizing the muscles and protecting the organs.

dorsiflexion: The motion of flexing the toes toward the shins.

extension: To increase the angle between body parts. This usually pertains to straightening a joint. The opposite of flexion.

external obliques: The muscles on the side of the midsection responsible for bending and twisting. These muscles work the same as the internal obliques, but the muscle fibers run the opposite direction.

external rotation: To rotate away from the center of the body. The opposite of internal rotation.

flexion: To decrease the angle between body parts. This usually pertains to bending a joint. The opposite of extension.

frontal plane: The plane of motion that separates the front and back halves of the body.

hamstrings: The muscle group in the back of the upper legs and thighs.

hip flexors: The muscles in the front of the body surrounding the pelvis that are responsible for flexing the hip joint.

hip joint: Composed of the femur and pelvis. Motions at the hip include flexion, extension, internal rotation, external rotation, adduction, and abduction.

internal rotation: To rotate toward the center of the body. The opposite of external rotation.

latissimus dorsi (lats): The large muscle group in the lower half of the back.

lumbar spine: The last 6 vertebrae of the spine.

pectoralis major (pecs): The muscle in the front part of the upper body that sits behind the breast tissue (the chest).

pectoralis minor (pecs): Another muscle in the front part of the upper body that sits behind the breast tissue (the chest). It assists the actions of the pectoralis major.

plantar flexion: The action of pointing the toes down and away from the shins.

quadriceps (quads): The muscle group in the front of the upper legs and thighs.

rectus abdominis: The "six-pack" muscle of the abdominals.

reps: The number of times one performs a movement in a set.

rhomboids: The upper back muscles that sit between the spine and shoulder blades. These are responsible for squeezing the shoulder blades together.

rotator cuff: The muscles that surround your shoulder blades and help stabilize the shoulder joint.

sagittal plane: The plane of motion that separates the left and right halves of the body.

scapula: The triangle-shaped bone that sits in the upper back (the shoulder blades).

sets: The number of times one repeats an exercise.

shoulder joint: The ball-and-socket joint created by the head of the upper arm and scapula. The actions of this joint are flexion, extension, internal rotation, external rotation, abduction, and adduction. It's the most mobile joint of the body.

superset: To quickly move from one exercise to another without taking a break in between the two.

thoracic spine (T-spine): The middle 12 vertebrae of the spine.

transverse abdominis: The most important muscle of the core. It protects the internal organs, regulates breathing, and stabilizes the spine.

transverse plane: The plane of motion that separates the upper and lower halves of the body.

trapezius (traps): The large muscle in the upper back that spans the back and tops of the shoulders.

triceps: The muscles in the back of the upper arm.

RESOURCES

Anatomy Trains, Thomas Myers: This book is a comprehensive resource on how fascia affects training.

ClassPass Go app: This app provides you with free strength workouts led by a trainer. One of those trainers is yours truly, Brittany Noelle.

Fitbod app: This app will create weightlifting programs for you based on your goals, muscle recovery times, and fitness level. It's very helpful while you learn the basics of programming.

Heart rate monitor: A heart rate monitor is a helpful tool for making sure that you are remaining in the correct training zone for your goals while you're working out. It is also very useful if you want to include cardio into your program.

MyFitnessPal app: This app is super helpful for tracking your food so that you can better understand how many calories you're consuming each day, as well as your macronutrient intake (protein, fat, and carbohydrates).

NASM Essentials of Personal Fitness Training, National Academy of Sports Medicine, Sixth Edition: This book is a great resource if you're interested in becoming a personal trainer, or if you're interested in learning more about programming and weightlifting.

Pocket Anatomy app: An in-depth and interactive way to explore human anatomy. You can see each system of the body and each individual muscle, including brief explanations of their functions and roles.

Precision Nutrition website: Precision Nutrition's nutrition coaching course and website (www.precisionnutrition.com) will help you have a better understanding of nutrition, specifically in relationship to health and fitness. Coaches teach a realistic, behavioral approach to nutrition.

Seconds app: This app will help you easily create timed workout sets. It's really helpful to keep you on track during your workouts.

Sleep Cycle app: Sleep is a very important part of recovery, which is key for weightlifting. You need to sleep in order to recover from your workouts properly. This app helps track how much sleep you've gotten and the quality of that sleep.

Strong-N-Fit blog: My blog is a useful resource for learning how to incorporate fitness into your lifestyle (www.bnoellefitness.com/strongnfit).

INDEX

ACKNOWLEDGMENTS

I want to thank my parents, Joy and Marvin Stalworth II, for paying for my expensive UCLA education and always supporting my dreams. Without my physiological science degree, I wouldn't know as much about the body as I do. I also wouldn't have fallen in love with weightlifting during my time running track and field. I also want to thank all the master trainers at various Equinox locations who have helped me become a better trainer and awesome at programming—especially Kori Lyn Angers. I also want to acknowledge some of the other amazing personal trainers at Equinox who have shared their fitness knowledge with me and helped me grow as a trainer: Special shout-out to my three best trainer friends, Billie White Muscarella, Lindsey Crosby, and Romina Denton. You're always there to support me, and I've learned so much from you all!

ABOUT THE AUTHOR

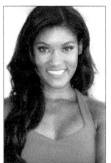 Brittany Noelle is a former Division I track and field athlete, World Beauty Fitness & Fashion (WBFF) champion, and contestant in Miss California USA. She is a National Academy of Sports Medicine (NASM) and National Council on Strength & Fitness (NCSF) certified personal trainer. Additionally, she is a certified health coach through the American Council on Exercise (ACE). She also holds certifications from TRX, Precision Nutrition, Pre/Postnatal, and Kettlebell Levels 1 and 2.

Brittany is a luxury personal trainer and offers customized online personal training programs for people all around the world. Her motto is "I do fitness that fits you." Her unique approach to fitness helps her clients fit fitness into their unique lifestyles, likes, and dislikes. Instead of making clients adhere to her training program, she creates a unique program that is tailored to each client. With this innovative approach, Brittany feels that her clients are much more likely to stick with their programs and reach their goals. She believes weightlifting and working out should always be fun and enjoyable.

When Brittany isn't training, she enjoys hanging out with her friends and family, and visiting Disney Parks and the Wizarding World of Harry Potter. (She's a Gryffindor—a Glytherin to be specific.) She also is a huge foodie and loves discovering new restaurants and cool bars. She believes that life is all about balance, mainly finding a healthy balance between working out and eating the things you love.

Printed in the USA
CPSIA information can be obtained
at www.ICGtesting.com
LVHW061652191023
761405LV00001B/5